Register Now fo
to Your

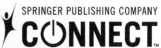

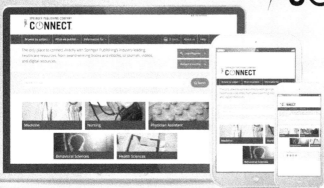

Your print purchase of *Conducting the DNP Project* **includes online access to the contents of your book**—increasing accessibility, portability, and searchability!

Access today at:

**http://connect.springerpub.com/content/book/978-0-8261-6837-5
or scan the QR code at the right with your smartphone
and enter the access code below.**

*Scan here for
quick access.*

> **94UCELAP**

If you are experiencing problems accessing the digital component of this product, please contact our customer service department at cs@springerpub.com

The online access with your print purchase is available at the publisher's discretion and may be removed at any time without notice.

Publisher's Note: New and used products purchased from third-party sellers are not guaranteed for quality, authenticity, or access to any included digital components.

SPRINGER PUBLISHING COMPANY

View all our products at springerpub.com

CONDUCTING THE DNP PROJECT

Denise M. Korniewicz, PhD, RN, FAAN, is the author of over 100 manuscripts and four books. She has held a variety of leadership, research, and faculty positions throughout her academic career. After receiving her degrees from Madonna University (BS), Texas Woman's University (MS), and the Catholic University of America (PhD), she completed postdoctoral education at the Johns Hopkins University, School of Nursing and the School of Medicine in the Department of Infectious Disease. She holds certificates in executive management and higher education from the Wharton School of Business, Carnegie-Mellon University, and Georgetown University, School of Nursing. She is a fellow in the American Academy of Nursing and has been awarded the American College of Clinical Engineering Challenge Award, the Georgetown University School of Nursing Faculty Award, and the mentor award for outstanding achievement from Sigma Theta Tau. Most recently, she has been presented with the Albert Nelson Marquis Lifetime Achievement Award by Marquis Who's Who.

Because of her research endeavors with interdisciplinary colleagues (microbiology, engineering, business, and biostatics), she has been a pioneer in the area of protective gear for healthcare personnel and has played a key role in the development of quality patient safety indicators, infection control standards, and international policies associated with new medical technologies. She has been recognized as a scholar, entrepreneur, business leader, and clinician.

Throughout her career, she has been instrumental in working with graduate students and has been a role model in both formal and informal healthcare organizations. Dr. Korniewicz's clinical research experience has provided multiple mentorship opportunities for DNP students. As a result of her extensive faculty, researcher, and administrative background, this book has been written to provide a practical approach for DNP students to develop their final DNP project. A step-by-step approach with specific examples as to how to successfully complete the DNP project has been provided.

CONDUCTING THE DNP PROJECT

Practical Steps When the
Proposal Is Complete

Denise M. Korniewicz, PhD, RN, FAAN

Editor

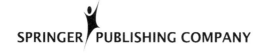

SPRINGER PUBLISHING COMPANY

Springer Publishing Company, LLC
11 West 42nd Street
New York, NY 10036
www.springerpub.com
http://connect.springerpub.com

Acquisitions Editor: Joe Morita
Compositor: Exeter Premedia Services Private Ltd.

ISBN: 978-0-8261-6826-9
ebook ISBN: 978-0-8261-6837-5
DOI: 10.1891/9780826168375

19 20 21 22 / 5 4 3 2 1

The author and the publisher of this Work have made every effort to use sources believed to be reliable to provide information that is accurate and compatible with the standards generally accepted at the time of publication. Because medical science is continually advancing, our knowledge base continues to expand. Therefore, as new information becomes available, changes in procedures become necessary. We recommend that the reader always consult current research and specific institutional policies before performing any clinical procedure. The author and publisher shall not be liable for any special, consequential, or exemplary damages resulting, in whole or in part, from the readers' use of, or reliance on, the information contained in this book. The publisher has no responsibility for the persistence or accuracy of URLs for external or third-party Internet websites referred to in this publication and does not guarantee that any content on such websites is, or will remain, accurate or appropriate.

Library of Congress Cataloging-in-Publication Data

Names: Korniewicz, Denise M., editor.
Title: Conducting the DNP project : practical steps when the proposal is
   complete / Denise M. Korniewicz, editor.
Description: New York, NY : Springer Publishing Company, LLC, [2020] |
   Includes bibliographical references and index.
Identifiers: LCCN 2019019656| ISBN 9780826168269 | ISBN 9780826168375 (ebook)
Subjects: | MESH: Education, Nursing, Graduate | Advanced Practice
   Nursing—education
Classification: LCC RT73 | NLM WY 18.5 | DDC 610.73071/1—dc23
LC record available at https://lccn.loc.gov/2019019656

Contact us to receive discount rates on bulk purchases.
We can also customize our books to meet your needs.
For more information please contact: sales@springerpub.com

Publisher's Note: **New and used products purchased from third-party sellers are not guaranteed for quality, authenticity, or access to any included digital components.**

Printed in the United States of America.

CONTENTS

CONTRIBUTORS

Maher M. El-Masri, PhD, RN, Wayne State University, School of Nursing, Detroit, Michigan

Denise M. Korniewicz, PhD, RN, FAAN, Wilkes University, Passan School of Nursing, Wilkes-Barre, Pennsylvania

Fabrice Immanuel Mowbray, MSN, RN, Department of Health Research Methods, Evidence, and Impact, McMaster University, Hamilton, Ontario, Canada

Carol Patton, DrPH, RN, FNP-BC, CRNP, CNE, Wilkes University, Passan School of Nursing, Wilkes-Barre, Pennsylvania

Maridee Shogren, DNP, CNM, University of North Dakota, School of Nursing, Grand Forks, North Dakota

Mary Wyckoff, PhD, RN, NNP-BC, ACNP-BC, FNP-BC, CCNS, CCRN, FAANP, Samuel Merritt University, School of Nursing, Sacramento, California

PREFACE

Once again, the education of primary care providers in the medical profession has resulted in a "call to action" by the Institute of Medicine (IOM, 2010) to increase the number of healthcare professionals who can provide care for the needs of an aging population. Advanced practice registered nurses are being used to provide the primary care manpower needs located in both rural and urban underserved areas. As a result of the increased need for advanced practice registered nurses, current changes in reimbursement patterns and the demographics in the United States, DNP programs are admitting the maximum number of graduate students and preparing them to be advanced practice registered nurses (National Organization of Nurse Practitioner Faculties [NONPF], 2016). In order to provide competent and safe advanced practice professionals, nursing programs often compete for faculty who have teaching and clinical experience and can provide mentored practicum experiences for enrolled students. However, due to the current faculty nursing shortage, most accredited nursing programs have to "cap" the number of students admitted to their advanced practice programs (American Association of Colleges of Nursing [AACN], 2015). As a result, most new faculty members lack faculty mentors, lack the teaching experience required in the classroom, and lack the skills necessary to provide learning experiences that are creative or innovative.

On the other hand, the DNP graduate student who returns to embark on graduate programs of study expect faculty to be well-rounded, knowledgeable, and have the ability to provide excellent mentored experiences. The DNP programs' course work is demanding and requires students to think independently, acquire clinical reasoning skills, and develop the clinical knowledge necessary to become safe advanced practice nurses. In order to meet these requirements, DNP faculty members develop a cadre of assignments that require the graduate to "think out of the box," provide evidence-based practice supportive documentation, and be able to develop written and oral skills consistent with the competencies required of a graduate student. Often, DNP students become frustrated with program faculty because they may be new to the faculty role, lack an understanding as to how to evaluate the student, and usually pull on their past clinical knowledge to mentor graduate students. All of these changes are demanding not only for the student but also for the faculty member. In fact, both faculty and students change as they move from semester to semester, and in the final semester, students begin to transition toward their final role as an advanced nurse practitioner.

One way to assist DNP students with the transition from beginning to program completion is to provide an assignment that makes the student combine all of their knowledge and clinical skills into one or two courses. These courses are identified in the DNP program as the "final DNP project." The final project allows DNP students to demonstrate to faculty their ability to integrate the basic science with the clinical sciences. The final DNP project is a clinical investigation into a clinical issue, such as improving the quality of patient care, providing more efficient healthcare services to a given population, changing clinical guidelines consistent with a clinical issue, or developing new ways to provide healthcare services to a population of patients. All of these projects require the DNP student to be knowledgeable about a clinical issue, use evidence-based scientific data, and be innovative by testing out their clinical idea.

The final DNP project helps students demonstrate their ability to lead change in the delivery of current and future healthcare. Often new faculty teaching in DNP programs as well as new DNP students are not sure how to begin their DNP project. In order to assist both DNP students and faculty members who teach in DNP programs, we have developed a book that provides the steps as to how to develop a DNP project. Faculty members often have differing perspectives as to what the DNP project should or could be, and students are not sure where to begin, what to include, how to work with different clinical staff, how to obtain institutional review, or how to defend what they write. As a result, we have provided a practical and logical sequence as to how to complete the DNP project. Each chapter has been written from the perspective of a new graduate DNP student or new faculty member who is beginning to teach in a DNP program. Specific content for each chapter has been provided with rationales and evidence-based content so that both the DNP student and a new faculty member can use the text to understand each content area.

Our approach differs from others in that we view the DNP project from the "eyes" of new graduate students or new faculty members teaching in the DNP program. The text begins (Part I) with an introduction to the clinical project, stages for implementation of the project, and the basics involved for submission to an institutional review board. Part II provides information about how to collect, analyze, and interpret the data consistent with the project. Part III includes how to work with the clinical staff, interprofessional collaboration, team building, and examples of debriefing all participants in the project. Finally, Part IV involves specific content related to the interpretation and dissemination of findings and how to contribute as a clinical scholar. As the reader progresses through the DNP program, we build on the knowledge, skills, and behaviors necessary to transition into an advanced practice nurse. Most importantly, there are examples as to how to include evidence-based practice approaches, how to successfully implement the project, and how to successfully defend the project to faculty, peers, and clinical partners. This approach assists both the DNP student and the faculty member to focus on the subject matter of the project and assists them in becoming a clinical scholar in their professional careers.

We believe that a well-written DNP project will provide the foundation for future clinical scholarship by DNP graduates. Future DNP graduates will become the future for clinical nursing practice. The DNP graduate will provide the clinical expertise needed within future healthcare systems. In fact, the DNP degree may become the future "entry into clinical nursing practice" licensure because of the technology and clinical expertise needed to provide population-based nursing care.

Therefore, the focus of this book provides the basis for understanding how to successfully implement and complete the DNP project. The tools provided within each section of the text assist the DNP student or new faculty member with lifelong learning skills that can assist in the transition from DNP student to future faculty member or clinical scholar. The examples associated with peer-review, scholarly writing, and publication have been presented so that DNP graduates and new faculty members can continue their careers beyond the scope of the DNP project.

The uniqueness of this book lies in its practical approach to completing the DNP project. The overall content is organized in a systematic and logical sequence for the development, implementation, and presentation of the DNP project. Both DNP students and faculty teaching in the DNP program will find this text useful since it clearly addresses the issues that DNP students encounter while enrolled in a program of study. Faculty teaching in DNP programs can use this book for DNP project courses or for faculty members to become familiar with DNP projects. Most importantly, by using the principles outlined for continued clinical scholarship, this book can be used by faculty teaching courses related to the DNP scholarly project as an orientation text for new DNP faculty members so that they can become familiar with student outcomes. Finally, this text may assist DNP faculty with the development of their own clinical scholarship.

REFERENCES

American Association of Colleges of Nursing. (2015). *The doctor of nursing practice: Current issues and clarifying recommendations. Report from the Task Force on the Implementation of the DNP.* Washington, DC: Author.

National Organization of Nurse Practitioner Faculties. (2016). *The doctorate of nursing practice clinical scholar: NONPF perspective.* Retrieved from https://cdn.ymaws.com/www.nonpf.org/resource/resmgr/docs/ClinicalScholarFINAL2016.pdf

Institute of Medicine. (2010). *The future of nursing: Leading change, advancing health.* Institute of Medicine Report. Washington, DC: The National Academies Press.

ACKNOWLEDGMENTS

The authors acknowledge the many individuals who have influenced the development of this book. The contributions from students and faculty to offer suggestions as to how to provide a practical approach to writing the DNP project have been most beneficial. We especially thank the faculty members who have discussed teaching strategies and have presented the examples used in the Application Exercises. We thank our families and friends for their ongoing support, patience, and encouragement as we worked on each section of this book. Finally, we thank our colleagues at Springer Publishing Company for assisting in the overall development of this text.

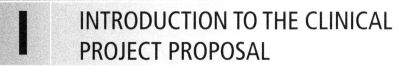

I INTRODUCTION TO THE CLINICAL PROJECT PROPOSAL

1 INTRODUCTION AND REVIEW OF THE CLINICAL PROPOSAL

DENISE M. KORNIEWICZ

INTRODUCTION

The American Association of Colleges of Nursing's (AACN) *DNP Essentials* (2006) has recommended that Doctor of Nursing Practice (DNP) projects should be the culmination of doctoral coursework and provide opportunities to translate knowledge into practice. The DNP project serves as the epitome of the practice-focused degree and provides the groundwork for future scholarship and meaningful contributions to improve nursing practice and patient outcomes. There may be a variety of clinical projects that may be represented including: quality improvement, healthcare policy, clinical-based inquiry, program development and evaluation, translation of evidence into practice, demonstration projects, or the generation of new evidence or knowledge (Brown & Crabtree, 2013). Regardless of the type of the DNP project developed, it must meet the minimum criteria suggested by the AACN (2006) and include the components of planning and evaluation.

Although the AACN has provided guidelines for the DNP project, faculty members continue to be dissatisfied with the outcomes of the DNP project (Dols, Hernández, & Miles, 2017). Reports in the literature (Dols et al., 2017; Embree, Meek, & Ebright, 2017; Nelson, Cook, & Raterink, 2013) classify faculty dissatisfaction with one of the following categories: (a) doctoral faculty attrition rates, (b) lack of faculty knowledge of evidence-based practice and quality improvement projects, (c) lack of clinical or university resources, and (d) lack of student's scholarly writing skills. On the other hand, chief nursing executives (Embree et al., 2017) identified DNP graduates as lacking the following skills: (a) system leadership, (b) science, and (c) translation of evidence into practice. In spite of these conflicting issues in academia and clinical practice, what remains important is that the DNP project investigates a clinical problem and includes the following components: purpose, project goals and objectives, project management, university and clinical requirements, quality management, project initiation plan, training plan, and required resources (AACN, 2006). This chapter begins with an already-established DNP project that has been developed. Keeping in mind that each DNP project may differ from one student to another, what is important is that the project has been logically developed and meets the DNP essentials (AACN, 2006). A step-by-step implementation phase has been outlined to assist individuals to logically move forward with the DNP project (Table 1.1).

TABLE 1.1 Implementation Phases for the DNP Project

Steps	Content	Action Steps
1	Review of official documents	IRB approval University signatures (advisors, faculty)
2	Assessment of proposal components (problem statement, review of literature, data methods)	Clinical problem to be investigated Review of the literature Data collection procedures Data analysis plan Outcomes
3	Presentation of proposal to clinical agency staff members	Presentation of general project Role of clinical staff Timeline for data collection Pilot phase Data collection phase
4	Making decisions or overcoming barriers	Understanding the clinical issues Providing feedback to clinical staff Reviewing data for accuracy Working with clinical staff to make any changes Obtaining input from faculty members and clinical staff
5	Presentation of the data analysis	Develop general overview of findings Provide findings Have further discussions with the clinical staff (what was good or bad) How would you change project if it completed a second time?

DNP, doctor of nursing practice; IRB, institutional review board.

The examination of the project will allow you to review the initial proposal and add or delete components that may have changed since the initial written proposal. The DNP implementation areas that are discussed include: (a) document review, (b) review of the proposal components, (c) presentation of proposal (orientation of clinical staff, data collection procedures), and (d) making decisions or troubleshooting while completing the overall goals of the project. Further examples of how to avoid barriers that may be encountered while completing the project are provided. A well-thought out and planned approach to implement the DNP project will assist in overcoming any obstacles that may occur during the project period. Thus, it is best to be prepared for any possible issue that may detract from the success of the project.

DOCUMENT REVIEW

One of the most difficult components of the development of the DNP project is getting started. A systematic approach to review each component of the proposal provides opportunities to make any changes that may impact the overall success of the project. This initial step includes review of all the documentation needed by your sponsoring clinical agency or university. Table 1.2 provides a list of the type of documents that may be required to initiate your project. Be sure all of your documents are up to date and have the appropriate signatures, dates, and approvals prior to initiating your project.

TABLE 1.2 Examples of Documents Required by the Clinical Agency or the University

Examples of Required Documentation	Clinical Agency	University
• Clinical agency approval to complete project (letter)	x	x
• IRB (proposal)	x	x
• University DNP committee members (signed document)	x	x
• Copyright approvals for use of any data collection tools	x	x
• Letter of approval from medical director (if applicable)	x	x
• Funding received (disclosure letter)	x	x

DNP, doctor of nursing practice; IRB, institutional review board.

REVIEW OF THE PROPOSAL COMPONENTS

The first and foremost area to review would be the problem statement. Be sure that it is clear and easily understood. Often the clinical problem statement is clarified by working with your faculty advisors and your peers so that it is distinct and provides an evidence-based statement that reflects a clinical situation.

The second area to review would be the review of literature or the evidence-based content that was used to support the project. One way to begin a review of literature would be to understand the importance of "essential" or "need to know" content versus literature that is not very important to your overall research question. "Need to know" content would be literature that specifically supports your project and highlights the dimensions of the problem (Waldrop, Caruso, Fuchs, & Hypes, 2014). Examples may include prevalence data or clinical outcomes or cost issues. Often when a review of the literature is used, the content may be more peripheral to the clinical question versus specific to the clinical question. This is a difficult task when learning to write the literature review. However, one way to edit a review of literature would be to evaluate the content that was initially proposed and describe the literature linkages that are relevant to the clinical area of study (Houser, 2015). Examples of a clearly defined literature review include the following:

- Description of the current status of the clinical question
- Consideration of content closely related to the clinical problem
- Identification of any gaps where one can argue that further clinical research is needed
- Explanation of how to plan to eliminate any gap in the literature.

Using a logical structure to review the need to know content of a clinical project assists in providing the important evidence-based literature available and provides a clear roadmap of how to examine the clinical question.

The second component includes the purpose and goals of the project. Usually, this is a straightforward statement about what the project will include. The review at this time is simply to be sure that all editorial changes have been made based on input from any committee members so that the purpose and goals are clearly written. Additionally, it is best to assess any changes in the wording or the purpose and goals based on any changes made during the final review of literature, changes at the clinical site, or changes related to any new clinical guidelines.

The third component includes the data collection methods and how the project will be implemented. The methods section is one of the most important components of the DNP proposal since each area needs to be well thought out and planned. Reviewing each component as to what, who, where, how, and the timeline that will be used for each step are all components of the implementation phase. At this stage, dissecting each area of the methods section will assist in carrying out the processes necessary to be successful.

For example, the data collection procedures need to be logically developed from beginning to end. One way to provide accurate information about the data collection procedures includes a data collection protocol that would be used to train any clinical staff or data collectors. This consists of a written protocol as to how the clinical staff or data collectors will be involved in the project. One approach that may clarify this process is to have a member of the clinical staff review the protocol and add or delete sections that may or may not be relevant to the process. This activity will help to clarify any discrepancies in the interpretation of the written protocol.

Writing down each step of the data collection phase will assist in providing consistent guidelines as to the overall reliability and congruence of the data collection (Howlett, Rago, & Gabiola, 2014). It is during this phase that a specific criterion is provided that relates to the process and time to "try out" the data collection tools. For example, if one is using electronic data collection tools, it is important that everyone knows how the data are collected, stored, and analyzed. If one is using paper and pencil, then the process for obtaining the data, storing the data, and reviewing the data should be part of the overall data collection criteria. Once the staff and data collection assistants are trained, then it is best to provide a pilot phase for data collection. The pilot phase may last 1 week or less and allows everyone to use the data collection tools, provide feedback as to what worked and what did not work, and allows time to modify the data collection procedures. Also, the pilot data collection phase provides the opportunity to make changes in the written protocol so that once the project is implemented, monitoring of the data collection is less challenging.

The fourth component of the methods section includes the development of a realistic timeline for presentation of the project, a training period for the clinical staff and data collectors, pilot data collection phase, data collection period, and analysis and results of the study. By reviewing each of these project components will assist in the development of the overall presentation of your project. For example, meetings associated with the clinical personnel for the data collection period requires a well thought out plan to inform the clinical staff. An in-service related to your data collection methods and introduction of your data collection staff would be an essential component to review during the implementation phase. It is best to provide a longer period of time for data collection so that the proposed number of events that were suggested as part of the initial proposal is met. The timeline helps clinical staff and research assistants understand the project as a whole and provides an overall roadmap of the project.

PRESENTATION OF PROPOSAL

The overall presentation of the DNP project should be clearly organized and address the purpose, goals, data collection, and outcomes of the project. A simple slide show or a 1-page handout with the essential content about the project will assist the clinical staff with the knowledge necessary to support the project. Topics that need to be addressed during the presentation include the role of the clinical staff member during the project period. Often, the clinical staff are concerned about the extra time involved to assist with the project. Because of workload concerns, it is recommended that the personnel needed to collect the data is provided versus relying on the clinical staff. What is important is to provide a clear, well thought out way in which the data assistants will be involved with the clinical staff. Figure 1.1 illustrates an example of how to develop an implementation plan for the clinical staff.

MAKING DECISIONS OR TROUBLESHOOTING

The final area to review in the implementation phase includes a checklist as to how one will intervene if an issue occurs while conducting

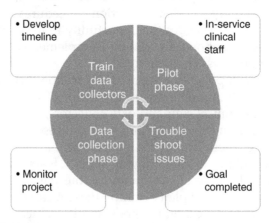

FIGURE 1.1 Project implementation for clinical staff.

the DNP project. Often problems that may arise include: (a) complaints from clinical staff or patients during data collection, (b) changes in the data collection timeline, (c) problems associated with peripheral issues such as the Institutional Review Board (IRB) or nursing managers who do not support the project, (d) lack of clinical staff support, (e) difficulty with data collectors (timeliness or dedication to project), (f) breech in data collection methods by clinical or project staff, or (g) a major change within the healthcare system itself that may impact the clinical area where the project is being conducted. Although it is not likely that anything may occur during the development of the implementation of the project, it is important to be prepared to troubleshoot any issues that may occur. Often one way to handle these issues include: (a) meeting with the faculty advisor(s) to assist with troubleshooting or suggestions, (b) meeting with the clinical manager or clinical support staff to assist with any resolution, (c) obtaining suggestions from other clinical experts who have had similar clinical problems and experiences, and (d) discussion with peers via a DNP clinical topics seminar. The more input as to how to prepare for any of issues that may occur during the DNP implementation phase will help to prevent any surprises and provide more positive outcomes when one is prepared to troubleshoot the problem. Thus, it is important to monitor each component of the DNP project beginning with the orientation of staff about the project, data collection phase, analysis of the data, and presentation of the results once the project is completed. The exemplar in Box 1.1 provides a realistic approach as to how to troubleshoot an unforeseen problem when implementing a DNP project.

Using a well-thought out implementation plan that reviewed all components of the DNP project will assist in the success of the DNP project. The implementation plan will help avoid any obstacles that may arise during the project phase. By following these recommendations, one can ensure the identification of any barriers or unforeseen problems that may occur. Thus, the value of the further development of the DNP project to include specifics related to any procedures, protocols, or monitoring plans will decrease any potential problems that may occur during the DNP project.

PRESENTATION OF THE FINDINGS

At this point, it is important that the clinical staff are informed as to the findings resulting from the project. It is best to mention this to the staff so that they are informed that you will present the findings once the project data collection procedures are completed. This will allow open

BOX 1.1 Monitoring and Troubleshooting Problems When Implementing a DNP Project

Ms. Mitchell reviewed her DNP proposal, provided an in-service to clinical staff, and began data collection procedures associated with quality improvement for post-op patients undergoing knee replacement. The post-op floor had 15 to 20 knee replacements per week, so the number of data points would not be an issue. Ms. Mitchell's data collection procedures included a 10-item patient satisfaction survey from patients as well as a 10-item clinical nursing staff assessment tool rating the intensity of the nursing care procedures. All of the data collection tools were electronic via the use of tablets for both the patients and the staff members. The key point in the data collection was the time period as to when the data were to be collected. The initial protocol required the clinical staff to obtain the data when the patient was ready for discharge. Ms. Mitchell provided a 2-day pilot data collection period and was pleased that the staff were "onboard" with the project. However, once the data collection phase was implemented, Ms. Mitchell noticed that she was getting incomplete data or no data at all after 1 week of the data collection period.

Example of DNP student intervention. Ms. Mitchell met with the clinical staff and found out that they often forgot to use the tablets that were provided since they were locked up at the nurse's station. Second, the staff were concerned that they would make an error in assisting the patient or when entering their own data. Third, patients were not familiar with using tablets, thus they refused to complete the questionnaire without help prior to their discharge time. After discussing the issues with the staff and her faculty advisor, Ms. Mitchell made the following changes to her data collection procedures:

1. Another in-service was provided to each shift, and clinical staff were provided with one-to-one hands-on teaching for the use of the tablets
2. Tablets were made available on the computer cart that was used for room-to-room nursing care
3. Clinical staff were instructed as to how to assist the patient during completion of the survey
4. Clinical staff were allowed to enter the patient's response for them if the patient had difficulty with the tablet

(continued)

BOX 1.1 Monitoring and Troubleshooting Problems When Implementing a DNP Project (*continued*)

---

5. Ms. Mitchell and her research assistant were available daily during the next 2 weeks to provide staff support
6. After the 2-week period, Ms. Mitchell provided a research assistant daily to be available to the clinical staff for any further instruction related to the use of the tablets
7. Ms. Mitchell provided the IRB and the clinical manager with a revision of the data collection procedures for her project

Resolution. Because Ms. Mitchell was actively monitoring the data collection process, she was able to quickly identify the problems and immediately intervene. As a result, she was able to successfully complete her project without any other issues. Thus, by planning out each step in the data collection process and immediately monitoring results of the data entries provided a proactive resolution for troubleshooting an issue that could have negatively impacted on the overall goals of the project.

---

conversations with the clinical staff and demonstrates the importance of their input. Further discussion and specificities about how to present the clinical findings can be found in Chapter 2, Stages for the implementation of the DNP Project.

SUMMARY

This chapter provided a logical outline as to how to implement the DNP project in the clinical area. Discussion included specifics associated with the DNP proposal such as review of the proposal components (problem, review of the literature, methods, or data collections procedures) and an understanding as to how to intervene if there are any issues that may occur during the project period. Finally, a presentation of the AACN's DNP essentials was provided to assure DNP students that the review components for the implementation phase of their scholarly project was consistent with national accreditation standards.

REFERENCES

American Association of Colleges of Nursing. (2006). *The essentials of doctoral education for advanced nursing practice.* Retrieved from http://www .aacnnursing.org/Portals/42/Publications/DNPEssentials.pdf

Brown, M. A., & Crabtree, K. (2013). The development of practice scholarship in DNP programs: A paradigm shift. *Journal of Professional Nursing, 29,* 330–337. doi:10.1016/j.profnurs.2013.08.003

Dols, J. D., Hernández, C., & Miles, H. (2017). The DNP project: Quandaries for nursing scholars. *Nursing Outlook, 65*(1), 84–93. doi:10.1016/j .outlook.2016.07.009

Embree, J. L., Meek, J., & Ebright, P. (2017). Voices of chief nursing executives informing a doctor of nursing practice. *Journal of Professional Nursing, 10,* 23–55.

Houser, J. (2015). *Nursing research: Reading, using, and creative evidence.* Burlington, MA: Jones & Bartlett Learning.

Howlett, B., Rago, E., & Gabiola, T. (2014). *Foundations of evidence based practice* (pp. 31–52). Burlington, MA: Jones & Bartlett Learning.

Nelson, J., Cook, P., & Raterink, G. (2013). The evolution of a doctor of nursing practice Capstone process: Programmatic revisions to improve the quality of student projects. *Journal of Professional Nursing, 29,* 370–380. doi:10.1016/j.profnurs.2012.05.018

Waldrop, J., Caruso, D., Fuchs, M. A., & Hypes, K. (2014). EC as pie: Five criteria for executing a successful DNP final project. *Journal of Professional Nursing, 30,* 300–306. doi:10.1016/j.profnurs.2014.01.003

CAROL PATTON

INTRODUCTION

This chapter focuses on an understanding of the contextual, programmatic, and healthcare issues that impact the development of a Doctor of Nursing Practice (DNP) project. Emphasis includes the plan, design, and evaluation of the DNP project. Strategies for how to implement the DNP project are described as well as information about the general principles of implementing the DNP project. Additional content will include information about data collection, monitoring, and evaluating the DNP project. Finally, strategies about how to manage the DNP project from beginning to end are presented.

FOCUS OF THE DNP PROJECT

The DNP is designed for nurses seeking a terminal degree in nursing practice and offers an alternative to research-focused doctoral programs. "DNP-prepared nurses are well equipped to fully implement the science developed by nurse researchers prepared in PhD, DNS, and other research-focused nursing doctorates" (American Association of Colleges of Nursing [AACN], 2017). Furthermore, the DNP is a degree that provides opportunities for innovation and collaboration in a variety of clinical and executive advanced practice roles (National Organization of Nurse Practitioner Faculties [NONPF], 2013, p. 1). For example, the DNP project can originate from a variety of foci including patient-centered care; healthcare systems at the micro-, macro-, and/ or meso-systems levels; population-focused care; and other areas that influence nursing directly or indirectly, including clinical practice gaps. Regardless of the DNP topic of interest, the essence of the DNP project is to improve healthcare quality and safety.

It is relevant to appreciate and be mindful that the ultimate role of the PhD-prepared nurse is to have knowledge, skills, and competency focusing on a research mission and generation of new knowledge (Hinton-Walker & Sperhac, 2009, p. 348). The ultimate role of the DNP-prepared nurse is to have a practice mission and apply the knowledge and science generated by the PhD-prepared nurse (Hinton-Walker & Sperhac, 2009, p. 348). Therefore, the differentiation between the PhD nurse and the DNP is essential when developing programs of study consistent with the Essentials of Doctoral Education for Advanced Nursing Practice (AACN, 2006).

Since the inception of DNP programs, there have been numerous titles for the DNP project. Because of the confusion associated with program outcomes, the DNP project has undergone a variety of proposed plans and designs. Box 2.1 indicates the various titles of final DNP projects that have been cited in the contemporary literature (Brown & Crabtree, 2013).

According to the AACN (2015), the current title for the culminating DNP product is a final DNP project. The final project should be called the "DNP project" to avoid confusion with the term Capstone, which is used at varying levels of education (NONPF, 2013). The DNP project is not a research dissertation; therefore, this term should not be used. There has been a clarion call and much debate between and among nurse educators and professional nursing organizations regarding confusion over the title of the DNP project. As a result of requests of clarity, the DNP final project has been entitled the DNP project (AACN, 2015; NONPF, 2013).

PROGRAMMATIC AND HEALTHCARE INFLUENCES

The *Essentials of Doctoral Education for Advanced Nursing Practice* (AACN, 2006) refers to the final DNP project (AACN, 2006) as an investigation into evidence-based practice health issues. As a result, there are multiple curricular models underpinning the DNP programs. Two examples of curricular models to achieve DNP degrees are BSN to DNP programs and post-master's DNP programs. DNP graduates regardless of the DNP curriculum must meet the DNP program outcomes. Regardless of the type of DNP program and curriculum,

BOX 2.1 Various Titles for DNP Projects

1. Research utilization project
2. Scholarly inquiry in nursing practice
3. Practice improvement project
4. Evidence-based mentoring applied project
5. Comprehensive study
6. Synthesis project
7. Scholarly leadership project
8. Advanced nursing project
9. Clinical immersion project
10. Translational research project
11. System change project
12. Advanced clinical project
13. Administrative project
14. Translational research scholarly
15. Initiative
16. Portfolio
17. Clinical scholarship portfolio
18. Clinical research
19. Capstone project
20. DNP project
21. Dissertation
22. Doctoral thesis
23. Clinical practice dissertation
24. Evidence-based project
25. Clinical inquiry project
26. Practice project
27. Leadership project
28. Scholarly project
29. DNP clinical project
30. Residency project
31. Scholarly Capstone project
32. Clinical Scholarship: Capstone
33. Clinical scholarship project
34. Doctoral project

DNP, doctor of nursing practice.

the expected outcomes need to demonstrate all of the competencies delineated in the DNP Essentials I through VIII (AACN, 2006). When considering the DNP project, DNP program outcomes should focus on two general categories: (1) roles that specialize as an advanced practice nurse (APN) with a focus on care of individuals, and (2) roles that specialize in practice at an aggregate, systems, or organizational level (AACN, 2006, p. 17).

DNP projects should focus on advanced practice nursing on any form of nursing intervention(s) that influence or shape healthcare outcomes for individuals or populations (AACN, 2015, p. 1). These nursing interventions include a variety of areas that underpin and guide the DNP project topic. The DNP "is an academic degree and is not a role" (AACN, 2015, p. 1). Rather, individuals completing a DNP degree help to influence and shape clinical outcomes for individuals or populations through *direct* or *indirect* care as an APN (Table 2.1).

TABLE 2.1 DNP Project Examples of Direct or Indirect Healthcare

Type of healthcare	Examples of DNP projects
Direct	Management of care for individual patients Management of care for populations Management of care for populations with special needs Management of care for vulnerable populations
Indirect	Nursing administration Executive leadership Health policy Informatics Population health

DNP, doctor of nursing practice.

KEY FACTORS THAT GUIDE THE DNP PROJECT

A key consideration that helps guide the proposed DNP project is to assess national healthcare topics and standards as well as professional nursing standards and/or clinical guidelines. For example, being familiar with contemporary topics that improve healthcare and patient outcomes provides excellent resources for DNP projects. Many DNP programs have students identify a proposed DNP project topic early in their program. The DNP program outcomes and DNP faculty advise students about project requirements and an acceptable DNP topic.

The DNP project topic is typically approved in collaboration with input from an assigned DNP faculty member or DNP Project Committee chair. The process for approval of the DNP project topic is typically described in the DNP program handbook. The DNP project faculty member is responsible for the ultimate oversight and guidance for mentoring the DNP student from beginning to end to complete the DNP Project.

DNP students often grapple with and struggle with their proposed DNP project topic. The DNP program also clearly outlines and depicts the process and guidelines for selecting an approved DNP project topic. A variety of healthcare quality organizations have provided a list of healthcare topics that are appropriate for DNP projects. Additionally, several healthcare organizations that impact and guide U.S. healthcare and healthcare quality for the 21st century have provided topics for DNP (Table 2.2).

Some of the common actual or potential gaps in direct or indirect advanced practice nursing roles to guide and shape DNP projects often relate to the eight DNP Essentials. One of the greatest challenges for DNP programs is to be certain that the DNP project is the same for all

TABLE 2.2 Selected Organizations That Impact and Guide U.S. Healthcare and Healthcare Quality for DNP Projects

Organizations	Web Site	Examples of U.S. Healthcare and Healthcare Quality Initiatives
National Academy of Medicine (NAM)	https://nam.edu/initiatives	Action collaborative on clinician well-being and resilience Global health risk framework Grand challenge for healthy longevity Human gene editing Vital directions for health and health care
Institute for Healthcare Improvement (IHI)	http://www.ihi.org	100 Million healthier lives Age-friendly health systems IHI leadership alliance The conversation project National Steering Committee for Patient Safety 5 Million lives campaign
The Joint Commission (TJC)	https://www.jointcommission.org/facts_about_the_joint_commission	• Emergency management • Health equity • High reliability • Infection prevention and control • Pain management • Patient safety • Sentinel event—sentinel event alert • Physical environment portal • Transitions of care portal • Workplace violence prevention
The American Nurses Association (ANA)	https://www.nursingworld.org	Nursing excellence Innovation and evidence Work environment
U.S. Department of Health & Human Services (DHHS)	https://healthfinder.gov/HealthTopics	Health topics A to Z
American Organization of Nurse Executives (AONE)	http://www.aone.org	Advancing academic progression in nursing education Research Workplace violence Hospital improvement innovation network
American Hospital Association (AHA)	https://www.aha.org	Advancing best practices for hospitals and health systems Promoting healthy communities Get involved

(continued)

TABLE 2.2 Selected Organizations That Impact and Guide U.S. Healthcare and Healthcare Quality for DNP Projects (*continued*)

Organizations	Web Site	Examples of U.S. Healthcare and Healthcare Quality Initiatives
Institute for the Future (IFTF)	http://www.iftf.org/home	Health + self research collection
World Health Organization (WHO)	http://www.euro.who.int/en/health-topics	Ebola virus disease Nipah virus infection Nutrition Hepatitis Top 10 causes of death • Nutrition home • Nutrition topics • Databases • Publications • Collaborating centers • Regional offices • About us Marketing of breastmilk substitutes: National implementation of the international code WHO plan to eliminate industrially produced trans-fatty acids from global food supply Public consultation on draft WHO guidelines: Saturated fatty acid and trans-fatty intake for adults and children Guidance to promote breastfeeding in health facilities Global nutrition monitoring framework: Operational guidance for tracking progress in meeting targets for 2025 • Feeding of infants unable to breastfeed directly in care facilities • Support for mothers to initiate and establish breastfeeding after childbirth • Creating an environment in care facilities that supports breastfeeding • Supplementary foods for the management of moderate acute malnutrition in children aged 6–59 months • HIV and infant feeding in emergencies: operational guidance The duration of breastfeeding and support from health services to improve feeding practices among mothers living with HIV • Fortification of rice with vitamins and minerals in public health

(*continued*)

TABLE 2.2 Selected Organizations That Impact and Guide U.S. Healthcare and Healthcare Quality for DNP Projects (*continued*)

Organizations	Web Site	Examples of U.S. Healthcare and Healthcare Quality Initiatives
		Guideline • UNICEF/WHO/The World Bank Group Joint child malnutrition estimates—levels and trends in child malnutrition • Protecting, promoting, and supporting breastfeeding in facilities providing maternity and newborn services: the revised baby-friendly Hospital Initiative 2018 Implementation guidance • Evidence-informed guideline development for WHO nutrition-related normative work: continuous quality improvement for efficiency and impact • Guideline: implementing effective actions for improving adolescent nutrition • Reducing stunting in children: equity considerations for achieving the global targets 2025
International Council of Nurses (ICN)	http://www.icn.ch	ICN advances nursing, nurses, and health through its policies, partnerships, advocacy, leadership development, networks, congresses, and special projects. • Events • Projects • Nursing policy • Advocacy • Education • Socio-economic welfare
U.S. Public Health Association (APHA)	https://www.apha.org	APHA works to improve access to care, bring about health equity, and support public health infrastructure. Public health is a broad field. We focus on the most important problems and solutions of our time: Chronic disease / Climate change / Communicable disease Community water fluoridation / Ebola / Environmental health Global health / Gun violence / Health equity Health in all policies / Health rankings / Health reform

(*continued*)

TABLE 2.2 Selected Organizations That Impact and Guide U.S. Healthcare and Healthcare Quality for DNP Projects (*continued*)

Organizations	Web Site	Examples of U.S. Healthcare and Healthcare Quality Initiatives		
		Healthy community design	Healthy housing	High school graduation
		Injury and violence prevention	Lead contamination	Maternal and child health
		Mental health	Preparedness	Prescription drug overdose
		Public health accreditation	Public health standards	Racism and health
		Reproductive and sexual health	School-based health care	Social determinants of health
		Substance misuse	Suicide	Tobacco
		Transportation	Vaccines	Zika

DNP, doctor of nursing practice.

graduates regardless of the type of DNP program. The DNP graduates should demonstrate the same skills and competencies related to the DNP project for BSN to DNP and post-master's DNP programs (AACN, *DNP Essentials*, 2006). Regardless of the type of DNP program, DNP faculty supervising and mentoring DNP students should have a clear understanding of the scope and influence that DNP projects have on the quality of patient care.

An important strategy is to make certain the DNP projects integrates a robust, comprehensive body of science that reflects current best practices and focus on the varying levels of evidence. The thematic underpinning for the DNP project should be on application of scientific evidence to ultimately improve scholarly practice (Patton, 2015). Examples of DNP topics can be found in Box 2.2.

A major concern to advance nursing science and improve health outcomes is to be certain that the DNP project is based on a strong scientific base and best practices. For example, it is unacceptable to generalize ideas from only one nurse and one experience when caring for one patient. DNP projects should include hierarchies of evidence ranging from case studies to randomized control studies. It is the strength of the scientific evidence reviewed that supports clinical practice change.

BOX 2.2 Examples of DNP Topics

1. Evidence-based practice change
2. Policy change in a healthcare organization at the micro-, macro-, or meso-system level
3. Program evaluation
4. Executive summary
5. Project evaluation
6. Quality and safety initiative
7. Procedure change
8. Evaluation of an innovative practice model
9. Clinical inquiry regarding a practice change
10. Systematic review of literature
11. Meta-analysis
12. Meta-synthesis
13. Interprofessional practice change
14. Patient education initiative to improve patient safety and outcomes
15. Worker safety initiative
16. Workplace violence prevention initiative

DNP, doctor of nursing practice.

There are a number of taxonomies to rate evidence and determine the strength of the scientific evidence. While DNP projects may vary from program to program, DNP students must have the knowledge, skills and competencies to conduct a review of literature, and grade the strength of the body of scientific evidence. For example, when apprais- ing the body of scientific evidence, the DNP student needs to exam- ine the Cochrane Collaboration of literature that consists of systematic reviews of randomized controlled trials (RCTs). DNP students should consider investigating not only nursing literature, but also reviewing comprehensive interprofessional research and best practices on their topic of interest.

One way to complete a comprehensive review of literature is to develop an evidence-based pyramid related to the topic. An evi- dence-based pyramid is a triangle with the base of the pyramid incorpo- rating the weakest level of scientific evidence. The weakest component is at the base of the pyramid with the highest level of scientific evidence found at the pinnacle of the pyramid. Each section of the pyramid demonstrates a level of scientific review. For example, the highest level of evidence consists of systematic reviews of RCTs. It is recommended that the student organizes the evidence-based scientific review by using an evidence pyramid as a guide for the project. This method will assist the student with a thorough and comprehensive review of the evidence-based science available for their DNP project (Figure 2.1).

DNP PROJECT: PLAN, DESIGN, AND EVALUATION

The evaluation process of any project should begin during the planning and design of the project. The DNP project needs to have two or three specific project goals or project outcomes written in a behaviorally measurable and time-specific manner. The successful DNP project has outcomes that are achievable, realistic, time-centered, and behaviorally measureable (Patton, 2015). Since many of the DNP projects must be completed in a relatively short period of time, the DNP project outcomes can be identified and refined in the planning phase of the DNP project. Waiting to determine how to evaluate the DNP project until after the implementation of results is inappropriate since how the project will be evaluated should be written as part of the DNP proposal. In addition, the DNP student should use valid and reliable measurement tools that evaluate the concepts, topics, and/or interventions that are under investigation.

Two of the most important aspects of an evidence-based project is to have a clear purpose and focused project outcomes that utilize valid and reliable measurement tools that help to achieve project goals (Newhouse, 2006, p. 110). It is relevant for nurses to focus on outcome measures that improve specific interventions and provide a "roadmap" for future generations (Whitman, 2004, p. 293). DNP project outcomes drive the methodology and strategies selected for the DNP project (Patton, 2015). These are the specific project goals that will be evaluated

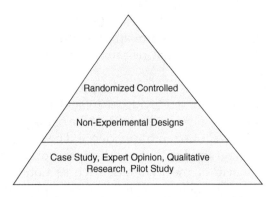

FIGURE 2.1 Scientific evidence pyramid.

to determine the success or failure of the project outcomes. Exhibit 2.1 provides an example of how to develop a DNP project that includes the problem statement, project outcomes, evaluation methods, and levels of measurement.

EXHIBIT 2.1 Example of a DNP Project

Exemplar

Effects of an Evidence-Based Educational Intervention to Increase Nurse Educator's Physical Activity at Work and at Home
      Despite the plethora of evidence and benefits of regular physical activity and exercise, many nurse educators do not engage in regular physical activity or, if they do, the level or extent of physical activity is insufficient to maintain a normal body mass index (BMI). Intellectually, nurse educators know better than anyone else why it is important to maintain a healthy body weight and have a normal BMI. BMI is the relationship of weight to height. For example, normal weight is a BMI between 18.5 and 24.9, underweight is a BMI under 18.5, overweight is a BMI from 24.9–30, and a BMI over 30 is obese. The purpose of this DNP evidence-based practice final project is to assess nurse educator's perceptions of exercise benefits and barriers on the Exercise Benefits/Barriers Scale (EBBS) before and after an evidence-based educational physical activity intervention.

NATURE OF PROJECT AND PROBLEM IDENTIFICATION

Significance of the Problem

Nurse educators are a population that may not get as much planned exercise and activity at work and at home as they need resulting in elevated BMIs. A BMI greater than 30 predisposes nurse educators to chronic health issues like chronic disease and illnesses like heart disease and stroke, respiratory problems, and muscle and joint problems. The purpose of this DNP Evidence-Based Practice (EBP) final project is to identify and assess perceived benefits and barriers of nurse educators to create a sustainable behavior change promoting increased physical activity at work and at home to keep the BMI within normal range.

The Problem

Many nurse educators are working in sedentary occupational roles presently. Nurses who complete fewer than 5000 steps per day are

(continued)

considered to have sedentary occupational sitting time (Munir et al., 2015). Nurses completing fewer than 5000 steps per day are at risk of preventable chronic disease and higher risk of increased mortality and morbidity from being overweight. For example, overweight nurses are more likely to experience poor health and chronic disease, resulting in higher absence from work, exit early from the nursing workforce, or take early retirement (Parry & Straker, 2013). Overweight nurses are also more likely to experience poor health and chronic disease, resulting in higher absence from work, exit early from the nursing workforce, or take early retirement (Parry & Straker, 2013).

Nurses serve as role models for patients and populations in many diverse healthcare settings. It is relevant for nurses to protect their health status with physical activity to maintain a normal BMI. Nurses, particularly nurse educators, cannot serve as role models to the patients/populations they serve unless they personally embrace and emulate the health status they are trying to impart to patients. For example, it is a challenge to talk with patients or populations about weight control and healthy BMI if the nurse is overweight. There is also an imperative for nurses working in sedentary roles in the workplace with respect to the nursing shortage. Nurse educators are a population of nurses who work in sedentary roles in the workplace. As more and more nurse clinicians and nurse educators assume sedentary occupational roles, the issues with obesity and limited physical activity as health risks will continue to increase, leading to more preventable chronic disease states that might have been prevented.

Project Outcomes

The five specific project outcomes for this DNP EBP final project are to:

1. Examine general levels of perceived benefits and barriers to exercise of nurse educators in a large urban College of Nursing regarding benefits and barriers to exercise (EBBS) pre- and post-evidence-based educational intervention.
2. Identify what nonexercising nurse educators perceived to be the biggest benefits of exercise.
3. Identify and assess what nonexercising nurse educators perceived to be the biggest barriers to exercise.

(continued)

4. Identify how nonexercising nurse educators perceptions of benefits from exercise are related to their perceptions of barriers to exercise.
5. Examine the impact (effect) of the evidence-based educational intervention on nurse educators pre- and post-intervention scores on the EBBS.

Plan for Evaluation of Data

This section provides an overview of the level of measurement on the EBBS, the statistical tests of analysis that will be computed using SPSS version 20, process for screening and cleaning data, how missing data, double answers, and other data problems will be resolved. It is essential for the DNP student to have a written plan for handling each of these issues, so the problem can be treated in the same manner and that there is a written record keeping a description of processes and outcomes of what was done to resolve these important research issues.

Level of Measurement

It is essential to use appropriate statistical techniques and statistical tests of analysis to analyze the quantitative data from the nurse educator's responses to the EBBS. The level of measurement of Likert scales is debatable as to whether Likert scales are ordinal or interval level data. The important concept is that the DNP student works with their DNP project faculty member or DNP committee chair and with a statistician during the DNP project planning phase to be certain the correct level of measurement of project outcomes with regard to selection of the measurement tool/measurement instrument like the EBBS is being used.

The reason scientific measurement of DNP project outcomes is essential is because the level of measurement greatly influences the scientific rigor of the DNP project by ensuring internal validity and reliability as well as generalizability of findings upon completion of the DNP project. Ordinal levels of measurement use categorical data, so the magnitude or range of data can be assessed. For example, if a nurse educator rates an exercise barrier as a score of 4, one cannot conclude that this nurse educator is four times more satisfied than a nurse educator who rates the same exercise barrier a score of 1. There is no true zero in ordinal level data. Without a true zero in

(continued)

ordinal level data, one cannot make inferences about the data from the project as the level of measurement is not at the interval level (Terry, 2015).

Using nonparametric tests are often referred to as *distribution-free tests* because they are based on assumptions. For example, nonparametric test do not assume that there is an equal or normal distribution (Terry, 2015). On the other hand, parametric tests do involve specific probability and assume normal distribution. Parametric tests assume the normal distribution and one would be examining whether or not the mean from the sample data is statistically significantly different than the mean of the parameters. Nonparametric tests will be utilized for this project based on the assumption that there is a normal distribution in the sample population for this DNP EBP final project. With the EBBS, the Likert scale is assumed to be interval level data and that the outcomes do follow a normal distribution.

EBP, evidence-based practice.

IMPLEMENTATION OF THE DNP PROJECT

Strategies and best practice for successful implementation of the DNP project require continuous monitoring and overview from beginning to end of the project. The DNP student should have a realistic timeline for completing the DNP project. Often, there are many key stakeholders and multiple dependencies that are often beyond the DNP student's control when completing the DNP project. For example, key stakeholders may go on vacation or become ill resulting in a delay in the progression of the DNP project. The clinical site where the DNP project is being conducted may experience issues that take precedence over the DNP project, causing delays in the DNP project. The DNP faculty mentor or DNP project chair may have untoward issues or setbacks resulting in delay of feedback to the DNP student. Typically, the DNP student should allow 7 to 10 business days for feedback from the DNP faculty mentor or DNP project chair. It is important to provide review documents to the DNP faculty mentor or DNP project chair in a timely manner and avoid any last minute completion of written documents (Patton, 2015).

The DNP student may not begin any implementation of the DNP project until Institutional Review Board (IRB) approval is obtained. Since there are multiple factors for the IRB approval process, DNP students will need to fully understand the required steps for IRB approval. Any changes or revisions to the approved IRB protocol must be amended and resubmitted to the appropriate IRB for review and re-approval. For example, if the DNP student determines that the DNP project will not be completed in the expected time period, the student will need to submit an amendment to the IRB with suggested changes in their project timeline.

The scope and logistics of the DNP project will need to be managed by the DNP student. The scope of the DNP project from start to finish is the ultimate DNP deliverable for completion of the project. A realistic timeframe for implementing the DNP project is typically 8 to 10 weeks. A delay in the DNP project timeline may interfere with the DNP student's plan of study and ultimately delay graduation. The DNP student must be familiar with DNP project policies and processes to fulfillDNP program outcomes and graduation requirements.

It is relevant for the DNP student to examine time and financial costs/expenses associated with the DNP project. For example, one cost associated with using measurement tools/instruments or surveys will need to be incurred by the student. Costs or permissions associated with measurement tools/instruments typically have an associated timeframe, so the DNP student will need to be certain that the timeframes are sufficient enough to complete the DNP project. By reviewing the timeline for use of any measurement tool will prevent the student from having to go back and add additional time as this may impact on IRB timelines, dates for completion, or university approvals.

One strategy to keep the DNP project on track is to use a timeline such as the Gantt chart (Gantt, 1910). It is highly recommended that the DNP student create a color-coded Gantt chart to monitor the DNP project timeline and progression from start to finish. The color-coded Gantt chart allows the DNP student to see at a glance if the DNP project is on time, falling behind, or moving forward toward completion. The Gantt chart is used as a DNP project-tracking dashboard to assist DNP students with any project issues that may delay or need additional support for successful completion of the overall project (Table 2.3).

COLLECTING AND MONITORING DATA

Strategies and best practice for collecting and monitoring data from beginning to end of the DNP project is the role and responsibility of the DNP student and faculty mentor. DNP programs have specific DNP project requirements for each component of the DNP project. Collecting and monitoring data from beginning to end of the DNP project will be clearly explained in the DNP project guidelines for each DNP program. The DNP student should focus on scientific best practices for each phase of the DNP project and adhere to the scientific principles that support the project.

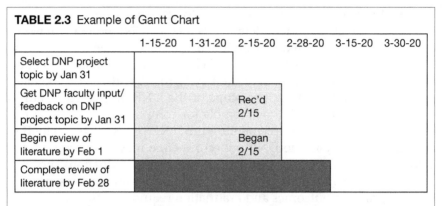

TABLE 2.3 Example of Gantt Chart

	1-15-20	1-31-20	2-15-20	2-28-20	3-15-20	3-30-20
Select DNP project topic by Jan 31						
Get DNP faculty input/ feedback on DNP project topic by Jan 31			Rec'd 2/15			
Begin review of literature by Feb 1			Began 2/15			
Complete review of literature by Feb 28						

1. Enter each DNP project activity/phase with a description and outcomes
2. Highlight each of the DNP project activities or phases to correlate to the timeline on the vertical access (by week, by month, and include the year)
3. Color code each of the DNP project activities or phases to correlate to the timeline on the vertical access (by week, by month, and include the year) using the following key:
4. Green (white) = on time and no issues
5. Yellow (gray) = nearly on time and project activity/phase is moving forward with few interferences or few dependencies on others to move the project to green status
6. Red (black) = There are major holdups and or issues and this activity/ phase is not moving forward or at a standstill/major impasse. This means that there are currently major threats to the project and high risk of not completing the project on time or more support is needed to move the activity/phase forward

Monitoring of data may seem like a simple thing to do; however, the DNP project requires that the DNP student manage the data from the beginning of the project to the end. The DNP student is accountable for all aspects of the DNP project including the IRB approval, data collection phase, final data analysis, interpretation of the results, discussion, and final presentation of the data. The DNP student must be certain that the DNP project data is collected in a scientific and rigorous manner so that there is no deviance from the data collection plan as set forth in the DNP project proposal. Additionally, all materials used for the project should be approved by the IRB without any substitutions.

Often, a DNP student may conduct his or her project at the current place of employment. As a result, the IRB may want the DNP student to have others known as a proxy or honest broker collect the data. The proxy or honest broker helps in the capacity of a research assistant to collect data, so there is no conflict of interest on the part of the DNP student. The DNP student is accountable for orienting and guiding the *proxy* or the *honest broker* to collect data in a scientific manner without deviation from the IRB protocol. Having a proxy or honest broker is often requested by IRBs when a DNP student is employed and currently working in the same facility where he or she is conducting the DNP project. The concept of using a proxy or honest broker avoids conflict of interest for the DNP student who is also an employee. Additionally, the DNP student should ensure that someone else is entering the data into the computer. This practice is to ensure that the DNP student remains objective about the data. However, monitoring the data entry process remains the task of the DNP student as well as any data cleaning, review for accuracy, missing data, and other data screening remain the responsibility of the DNP student.

It is essential that the DNP student acknowledges that there cannot be any deviation of the data collection tools or data collection protocol once all materials have been IRB approved. If changes occur as a result of clinical practice changes or errors associated with the initial written materials that were submitted to the IRB, the DNP student must inform the faculty members and collaborate with their faculty member to submit a revised IRB protocol and wait for approval of the changes prior to proceeding with the DNP project. It is best to work collaboratively with their DNP faculty mentor and the healthcare organization with the most detailed and approved IRB protocol for the DNP project. There cannot be any deviations from the approved IRB approval letter. Finally, the IRB approval letter should be submitted in its original form as an appendices with the final written DNP project.

MANAGEMENT OF THE DNP PROJECT

Managing and overseeing the DNP project for a successful DNP project from start to finish is demanding, time-consuming, and labor-intensive. There is no room for marginal or erroneous work when completing the DNP project. The DNP project embraces each DNP program outcome or DNP program goal. The final DNP project is a scientific process exemplifying that the DNP student has the knowledge, skills, and competencies to meet the eight DNP essentials (AACN, 2006).

Successful management and oversight of the DNP project takes perseverance, interprofessional collaboration, communication, ability to meet deadlines, ability to accept peer feedback, and criticism to have a scientifically rigorous scholarly product that can be disseminated externally to larger audiences. The ultimate goal of the DNP project is to have a final project that demonstrates clinical scholarship (NONPF, 2016, p. 3).

The DNP student will be stretched in his or her thinking when completing the final DNP project since it will involve multiple iterations and drafts. The DNP student should expect and welcome feedback and comments from peers, faculty, or clinical experts who provide feedback on multiple drafts. Scholarly writing is a challenge for many DNP students as typically nurses are not accustomed to scientific writing or are they used to providing evidence-based support for their ideas. Some DNP programs offer extensive editing services and scholarly writing support to DNP students but that is not always the case. Some DNP students are encouraged to have professional editing done at their own expense to complete a scholarly document within the designated DNP project timeline. Ultimately the DNP project should culminate in a publishable scholarly document that can be disseminated to wider audiences external to the DNP program.

SUMMARY

This chapter focused on the understanding of the context, programmatic, and healthcare issues that impact the development of the DNP project. Emphasis included the plan, design, evaluation, and management of the DNP project. Strategies for how to implement the DNP project were described as well as information about how to collect and monitor data. An example of how to write a DNP proposal abstract (Exhibit 2.1) was provided to assist students with formatting and writing a DNP proposal. Finally, additional content in this chapter included the importance of IRB approval and the process for collaborating with faculty members and other health professionals during the extent of the project.

REFERENCES

American Association of Colleges of Nursing. (2006). *The essentials of doctoral education for advanced nursing practice.* Retrieved from http://www.aacnnursing.org/Portals/42/Publications/DNPEssentials.pdf

American Association of Colleges of Nursing. (2015). *The doctor of nursing practice: Current issues and clarifying recommendations. Report from the Task Force on the Implementation of the DNP.* Washington, DC: Author.

American Association of Colleges of Nursing. (2017). *Fact sheet: The doctor of nursing practice (DNP).* Washington, DC: Author.

Brown, M. A., & Crabtree, K. (2013). The development of practice scholarship in DNP programs: A paradigm shift. *Journal of Professional Nursing, 29,* 330–337. doi:10.1016/j.profnurs.2013.08.003

Gantt, H. L. (1910). Work, wages and profit. *Engineering Magazine.* New York, NY; republished as Work, Wages and Profits. Easton, PA: Hive Publishing Company. Retrieved from www.gantt.com and What is a Gantt Chart?

Hinton-Walker, P., & Sperhac, A. M. (2009). The DNP and unintended consequences: An opportunity for dialogue. *Journal of Pediatric Health Care, 23*(5), 348–350. doi:10.1016/j.pedhc.2009.06.004

Munir, F., Houdmont, J., Clemes, S., Wilson, K., Kerr, R., & Addley, K. (2015). Work engagement and its association with occupational sitting time: Results from the Stormont study. *BMC Public Health, 15*(3), 1427–1439. doi:10.1186/s12889-015-1427-9

National Organization of Nurse Practitioner Faculties. (2013). *Population-focused nurse practitioner competencies: Family/across the lifespan, neonatal, acute care pediatric, primary care, pediatric, psychiatric-mental health, & women's health/gender-related care.* Retrieved from https://www.pncb.org/sites/default/files/2017-02/Population_Focused_NP_Competencies.pdf

National Organization of Nurse Practitioner Faculties. (2016). *The doctorate of nursing practice clinical scholar: NONPF perspective.* Retrieved from https://cdn.ymaws.com/www.nonpf.org/resource/resmgr/docs/ClinicalScholarFINAL2016.pdf

Newhouse, R. P. (2006). Selecting measures for safety and quality improvement initiatives. *Journal of Nursing Administration, 36*(3), 109–113. doi:10.1097/00005110-200603000-00002

Parry, S., & Straker, L. (2013). The contribution of office work to sedentary behavior associated risk. *BMC Public Health, 13*(1), 1–10. doi:10.1186/1471-2458-13-296

Patton, C. M. (2015). The impact of DNP projects on quality and safety in health care organizations. In B. Anderson, J. Knestrick, & R. Barroso (Eds.), *DNP Capstone projects: Exemplars of excellence in practice.* New York, NY: Springer Publishing Company.

Terry, A. J. (2015). *Clinical research for the doctor of nursing practice* (2nd ed.). Burlington, MA: Jones & Bartlett.

Whitman, G. (2004). Nursing sensitive outcomes in cardiac surgery patients. *Journal of Cardiovascular Nursing, 195*(5), 293–298. doi:10.1097/00005082-200409000-00003

3 INSTITUTIONAL REVIEW BOARD PROCESS AND THE DNP PROJECT

CAROL PATTON

INTRODUCTION

This chapter focuses on the requirements for the Institutional Review Board (IRB) process and the DNP project. This chapter includes the following: (a) an overview of the history of the IRB; (b) strategies and considerations for writing an IRB application specific to the organization granting IRB approval; and (c) the types of IRB reviews. Specific emphasis includes issues about IRB approval and vulnerable populations. Additional content discusses topics and concepts about: (a) the purpose and focus of the IRB pertaining to the DNP project; (b) definition of human subjects; (c) creating a realistic timeline for the IRB application; (d) working with de-identified data; (e) understanding the IRB submission and approval process; (f) obtaining permissions for tools/measurement instruments; (g) understanding the need for adhering to the approved IRB protocol; and (h) completing follow-up reports to the IRB upon completion of the DNP project. This chapter emphasizes the role of the IRB and oversight of ethical, principled research protecting human subjects involved in DNP projects.

OVERVIEW OF IRBs

The impetus for IRBs came about as a result of the research atrocities committed by the Nazi regime during World War II. These research violations and atrocities resulted from the Nazi regime performing unethical research on human beings. The research on human beings was so unethical and unprincipled that the behaviors resulted in trials and punishment for those committing the heinous crimes with what is now known as the Nuremberg Trials.

The Nuremberg Trials were held in Nuremberg, Germany, in December 1946 (Ingham-Broomfield, 2017). The purpose of the Nuremberg Trials was to hold those responsible for the heinous research on human subjects who could not protect themselves. The Nuremberg Trials resulted in creation of seven Nuremberg Principles that would protect human subjects involved in research and prevent these atrocities from being repeated. The seven Nuremberg Principles became known as the Nuremberg Code, which now guides all research involving human subjects (Ingham-Broomfield, 2017).

Although the Nuremberg Trials attempted to eradicate all future unethical research on human subjects, an example of immoral and unethical research known as the Tuskegee Syphilis Study was conducted in the United States in 1932 (Ingham-Broomfield, 2017). This study was conducted by the U.S. government on vulnerable African American men and consisted of research studying syphilis. There was a control group and a treatment group of poor, African American men known to have syphilis. The control group did not receive the drug, penicillin, known to cure syphilis in 1947 and the experimental group received penicillin. Treatment was deliberately withheld for the control group of men with syphilis, and the results were horrendous for those men left untreated. The results of this immoral research were so catastrophic that even today, there is still mistrust regarding research by many in the African American population (Perrin, 2014).

Another key document focusing on human research subjects' protection was *The Belmont Report. The Belmont Report* (1979) was released by the National Commission for the Protection of Human Subjects of Biomedical and Behavioral Research (1979). This report provided the ethical framework for the U.S. federal regulations for the protection of human research subjects. *The Belmont Report* includes the basic ethical principles that underpin biomedical and behavioral research when human subjects are involved in research. Even with documents like *The Belmont Report*, it is still necessary to have IRBs review all research protocols including DNP projects.

It is relevant to review the history and origins of IRBs and understand the role of the DNP student in human subject protection while working on the DNP project. The events and documents leading to ethical principles underpinning ethical and moral research cannot be overly emphasized. DNP projects require oversight in order to protect human subjects involved in any activities associated with patient outcomes or any review of data within health systems that track the quality of patient care.

IRB APPROVAL, PROCESS, AND THE DNP PROJECT

An IRB provides oversight and monitoring of the ethical, moral, and scientific integrity of every research project conducted in an organization or institution. The purpose of the IRB is to provide oversight of research involving human and animal subjects. IRBs review and approve all research activities involving human subjects to ensure that the research is conducted in accordance with all federal, institutional, and ethical guidelines.

IRB committees typically comprise internal and external members to the organization. For example, in an academic institution (college or university), the IRB comprises faculty members who have a research trajectory and knowledge of the research, scientific process, and ethical principles of research involving human subjects. There may also be a member of the clergy, a lay member from the community, and a member with a background in ethics and/or philosophy. The IRB committee membership is composed of key stakeholders with educational and experiential knowledge, skills, and competencies who determine if all research projects adhere to the ethical and principled human subject protection required in the research protocols before, during, and after the research project is conducted.

The IRB is tasked with assessing the proposed research protocol to ensure human subject protection. The IRB usually consists of members knowledgeable and aware of the processes used to assess if the proposed human subject research poses threats to human subjects (Biros, 2018). A common misconception of DNP students is that the DNP project does not involve any threats or risk to human subjects. For example, DNP students commonly have the misperception that if they are working on a quality improvement DNP project, they do not need IRB approval. The reality is that all types of DNP projects need to be reviewed to ensure that individuals who are involved in the research process are protected.

A human subject is defined by federal regulations as "a living individual about whom an investigator conducting research obtains (a) data through intervention or interaction with the individual, or (b) identifiable private information" (U.S. Department of Health and Human Services [DHHS], Office of Human Research Protection [OHRP], 45 CFR 46.102(f) 2018). All DNP projects must be submitted to the IRB for review and approval prior to implementing or conducting the DNP project. This includes a DNP project using de-identified data or one that focuses on the integration of evidence and best practice into a policy or practice change in a healthcare setting.

It is essential for the DNP student to recognize that human subjects may participate in a DNP project study in multiple ways. For example, a human subject may be actively involved in a DNP project by direct engagement such as responding to a survey face to face, being interviewed by the DNP student, or through responding to a questionnaire in an emailed survey. Human subject data may be accessed and collected from retrospective medical record review, via review of open public records, review of de-identified data sets, and/or through quality improvement projects. Box 3.1 provides examples of DNP project documents that should be included for IRB review.

TYPES OF IRB REVIEWS

DNP projects may warrant different types of IRB review. For example, there are typically three major types of IRB reviews: *exempt*, *expedited*, and *full board review*. Box 3.2 provides characteristics of each of the three major types of IRB reviews that the DNP student needs to be familiar with when completing the DNP project IRB application. The type of IRB

BOX 3.1 Examples of DNP Project Documents for IRB Review

1. DNP project protocol(s)
2. Written informed consent form(s)
3. Subject recruitment procedures (e.g., posters, emails, advertisements, or scripts for radio ads)
4. Written information to be provided to subjects (e.g., questionnaires or subject diaries)
5. Investigator's brochure
6. Informed consent form
7. Information about payments and compensation to subjects
8. Overview and brief information regarding the DNP student and this particular DNP project with a current curriculum vitae
9. Each IRB may request additional documents depending on the type of IRB review
10. Amendments if needed or if requested

IRB, Institutional Review Board.

BOX 3.2 Characteristics of the Three Major Types of IRB Reviews

Exempt

A research activity is typically exempt if it is considered low risk to the subject. Exempt categories for DNP projects are outlined in federal law 45 CFR 46.101(b).

Examples of categories for DNP Projects considered low risk are:

1. DNP projects conducted on education focusing on educational strategies and/or practices
2. DNP projects using anonymous surveys, interviews, or observations that cause no physical or psychological harm or risk
3. DNP projects that focus on collecting or studying existing data if publicly available or if working with de-identified data that cannot be linked to human subjects in any way
4. DNP projects evaluating policy, procedures, and/or program evaluation

Expedited

A DNP project may qualify for expedited review if it is determined that the proposed DNP project involves minimal risk, does not include intentional deception, does not employ sensitive or vulnerable populations or topics, and includes appropriate informed consent procedures and informed consent forms. Examples of DNP projects meeting criteria for expedited review include:

1. Collection of data from voice, video, digital, or image recordings
2. DNP projects focusing on individual or group characteristics or behavior (including, but not limited to, research on perception, cognition, motivation, identity, language, communication, cultural beliefs or practices, and social behavior), or projects using surveys, interviews, oral history, focus groups, program or project evaluation, human behavior evaluation, and/or quality improvement and evidence-based DNP project designs
3. Collecting physical data through noninvasive procedures. For example, computing the basal metabolic index, height and weight of subjects; MRI, EKG, ultrasound; moderate exercise; collection of blood samples by heel stick or finger stick. (See a full list of procedures at 45 CFR 46.110.)

(*continued*)

BOX 3.2 Characteristics of the Three Major Types of IRB Reviews (*continued*)

Full Board

A full board review is conducted when the DNP project involves more than minimal physical and/or psychological risk, involves protected, vulnerable populations including children, prisoners, or disabled individuals. Full board reviews occur typically on a timeline published well in advance so that DNP students are aware of the due dates for submission of applications well in advance.

Examples of DNP projects requiring full board review include:

1. DNP projects for which the level of physical and/or psychological risk is determined by the IRB Chair to be more than minimal
2. DNP projects involving intentional deception of subjects in a manner that is misleading or untruthful information is or could be provided to subjects
3. DNP projects involving protected, vulnerable populations including children, prisoners, or disabled individuals
4. Projects that plan to use procedures having the potential to be personally intrusive, stressful, physically or psychologically invasive, or potentially traumatic in some manner.

IRB, Institutional Review Board.

review for the DNP project determines the length of time it will take to obtain IRB approval and begin the DNP project. The DNP student may not begin implementing the project until written IRB approval is obtained from the IRB.

It is important that DNP students understand and embrace the type of IRB review needed for their specific DNP project while they are planning and designing their DNP project topic. The DNP student needs to understand the *Code of Federal Regulations* (Title 45 CFR) with respect to which types of reviews are needed for their DNP project. It is best to review the decision charts provided by the OHRP prior to IRB submission to ensure that the appropriate procedures are followed (DHHS, OHRP, 2018). The *Code of Federal Regulations* known as Title 45 CFR, Part 46.102.f is located on the website of the OHRP. Box 3.3 provides decision

BOX 3.3 Human Subject Regulations' Decision Charts

The OHRP provides excellent graphic aids that serve as decision guides for IRBs, investigators, and others who decide if an activity is research involving human subjects that must be reviewed by an IRB under the requirements of the U.S. Department of Health and Human Services regulations at 45 CFR part 46. These human subject decision charts help the DNP student address decisions regarding:

- Whether an activity **is research** that must be reviewed by an IRB
- Whether the review may be performed by **expedited procedures**
- Whether **informed consent** or its documentation may be waived

IRBs, Institutional Review Boards; OHRP, Office for Human Research Protections.

Source: From U.S. Department of Health and Human Services. (2016). Human Subject Regulations Decision Charts. Retrieved from https://www.hhs.gov/ohrp/regulations-and-policy/decision-charts/index.html

charts that will assist the DNP student with knowledge about how to address decisions regarding human subjects.

INFORMED CONSENT

Informed consent means the person involved in a research project of any type has the right to know what happens to their personal data from their medical records (Biros, 2018). Every research subject must be given the opportunity to say whether or not he or she consents to be a participant in the DNP project. The IRB application makes certain that the researcher has clearly described every detail with respect to how the research subject is made aware of the research project and has consented based on the ethical rights of research subjects and that no harm has been caused by minimizing research risks.

Informed consent is obtained based on the decision-making capacity of research subjects. Decision-making capacity to provide informed consent to participate in a research study is the ability of the research subject to understand what the project entails and to decide if he or she wants to participate in the research study. The process of obtaining informed consent in the IRB application must be detailed enough to prevent research-related harm, provide respect and individual autonomy to the research participant(s), and ensure that the burdens, risks, and potential harms from the research are equally and fairly distributed between and among research participants (Biros, 2018). For example, the IRB committee must be convinced that the researcher has clearly identified the type and nature of research activity that will be conducted and the actual and/or potential threats to the research and has clearly described these to the research participant.

Informed consent must be focused on the decision-making capacity of the research subject over time. Over time, decision-making capacity of the research subject may change or fluctuate; that is why the IRB research application must include the original signed actual research participant's consent form. There must be a statement in the informed consent form that tells research participants that they have the right to withdraw from the research study at any time without fear of retribution or harm if they change their minds about participation in the research study. For example, a person's decision-making capacity to participate in or consent to be a research participant may change based on a new life stressor, an illness, or a move to another town.

While obtaining informed consent may appear straightforward, there is also a specific process the DNP student must follow in documenting informed consent for the DNP project. The key concepts for documenting that the federal guidelines meet the IRB requirements' informed consent include the decision-making capacity, age, mental status, and overall understanding of the research project by the participants. Documentation of informed consent is an essential component of any DNP IRB procedure and must be adhered to in order to meet all federal guidelines.

Assent Versus Consent

It is important for the DNP student working with children or minors to understand the concepts of assent and consent. It is particularly relevant for the DNP student to understand who cannot give consent in order to understand the concept of *assent*. The term assent is used to express the willingness of a person under the age of 18 years old to participate in a research study (Al-Sheyab, Alomari, Khabour, Shattnawi, & Alzoubi, 2019). While assent is not legally binding, it is important in research to include children and/or minors less than age 18 by asking the child and/or minor if he or she wishes to assent or dissent from the decision. The rationale is that as researchers, DNP students should include children and/or minors less than age 18 out of respect for them as developing adults. The focus of the assent process in research is that children and/

or minors less than age 18 should be engaged in their health and life decisions because they will become adults caring for themselves as they assume responsibility from their parents (Baines, 2015). DNP students should understand the similarities and differences among assent, consent, and parental permission when the DNP project involves children and/or minors less than age 18.

The assent process involves an explanation to the child and/or minors less than age 18 regarding specific processes and components of the DNP project. For example, the assent process should provide information to the child and/or minor less than age 18 regarding the focus of the DNP project, why the project is being conducted, what the intervention will be, and how to withdraw from the project. Specifically, the child and/or minors less than age 18 must be informed and understand that they can withdraw from participating in the project at any time without fear of punishment, negative impact on their medical care, and or fear of retribution.

When children or minors (<18 years of age in many states, including Virginia) are involved in research, the regulations require the assent of the child or minor and the permission of the parent(s) in place of the consent of the subjects. The IRB guidelines will provide details and specificity for DNP students regarding assent versus consent when the DNP project involves children. Factors that are included when obtaining assent versus consent include the focus of the DNP project, age, health status, decision-making capacity, mental status, and parental relationships. What is relevant to consider is whether or not assent is needed and when to obtain permission of assent in DNP projects. For example, it is not essential to engage children and/or minors less than age 18 in assent when the research may not benefit the subjects. However, it is may be essential to engage children and/or minors less than age 18 in assent when the research is an important topic and of particular value and when the subjects have the decision-making capacity to understand what it means to be involved in research that benefits others.

IRBs determine what tools are acceptable to use in obtaining informed consent or assent. The IRBs have very detailed protocols and typically an example available for responding if/when issues arise about the DNP project. For example, if a subject does not appear to fully understand the project and the DNP student assesses the subject who appears confused about the project, there is guidance and support from the IRB regarding actions to take to protect the human subject. There is always contact information included in the consent or assent form as to who to contact if the subject or guardian has any questions at any time regarding the project. This contact information typically includes the DNP student, faculty member or chairperson, as well as the IRB office information.

DNP STUDENT PREPARATION FOR IRB AND ETHICAL RESEARCH

The majority of DNP programs have a course, the Collaborative Institutional Training Initiative (CITI, 2018), which DNP students must complete. The focus of CITI is to prepare the DNP student regarding human subject protection. The CITI program is offered as web-based training through the University of Miami. The CITI program consists of courses written and developed by peer-reviewed research experts. The university that the DNP student is attending specifies which CITI modules the student must complete for the training. In the event that the university does not specify which CITI modules the student must complete, the DNP student should check with their DNP faculty or chair or with the university IRB contact person. Typically, completing the required CITI training program modules takes on average of 10 to 15 hours. Students can save the completed modules and resume working on them at a future time. The CITI Training Program website is located at about.citiprogram.org/en/homepage.

Commonly Required CITI Modules

Commonly required CITI modules are Responsible Conduct of Research (RCR) and Good Clinical Practice (GCP). RCR consists of a basic course in ethical conduct of research but expands on several concepts and topics. GCP includes basic courses in ethical conduct of different types of clinical research. The RCR and GCP modules consist of reading and reviewing content focusing on key research concepts and topics for conducting ethical and principled research, reviewing key concepts and topics in the module, and completing a quiz at the end of each module. After taking the quiz at the end of each CITI module, quiz results and quiz scores are immediately available. The passing score for each quiz is 80%. One may go back and review content in the module and retake the quiz to obtain a higher score if/when scoring is less than 80% on a quiz. There are a variety of numbers of quiz questions in each CITI module, with some quizzes having as few as three questions and others having as many as 12. Finally, it is essential that one's CITI training is up to date and current in order to receive IRB approval, collect data, and complete the DNP project.

DETERMINING WHICH IRB TO SUBMIT THE DNP PROJECT

It is essential that DNP students examine their university or healthcare organization to know the specific IRB guidelines and regulations required for the setting where the study will be conducted. Many university and colleges have a Letter of Agreement or Letter of Determination process allowing DNP students to submit their DNP project to the IRB in the setting where the DNP project will be completed. For example, some DNP students carry out their DNP projects in the hospital or healthcare settings where they work. Therefore, the DNP students would submit their DNP project according to the IRB requirements of their hospital or healthcare setting where they work. Once IRB approval is obtained from their hospital or healthcare setting, then they would submit the Letter of Agreement or Letter of Determination to their university or college IRB. Once the Letter of Agreement or Letter of Determination is recognized by the university or college IRB, the DNP students can begin implementing their DNP project.

VULNERABLE POPULATIONS

There are additional protections needed for selected subjects for DNP projects that include pregnant women, fetuses, neonates, prisoners, children, and persons with disability and/or mental health issues. These subjects are considered vulnerable populations or selected populations. Box 3.4 provides examples of vulnerable populations that have been considered by IRB boards. DNP students completing their DNP project need to be aware that working with vulnerable populations will most likely include a full Board review taking more time than a DNP project that is an exempt or expedited review. Regardless of the patient population of study, DNP students should manage their time appropriately to include IRB approval.

BOX 3.4 Sources of Vulnerability Related to Research Projects

- Being a member of a specific group like a racial minority or group that is socioeconomically deprived
- A member of a vulnerable group: women, racial minority, fetuses, neonates, prisoners, children, persons with a disability or mental health issue
- Having a personal characteristic like being in a subordinate position to the DNP student because the student is the supervisor of the research subject(s)
- A DNP project is poorly designed increasing the risk of harm
- Lack of needed detail and specificity in the consent form

(continued)

BOX 3.4 Sources of Vulnerability Related to Research Projects (*continued*)

- Language is used during explanation of the consent form and DNP project that is above the educational level of the research subject making him or her vulnerable to lack of understanding
- Stigma and shame resulting from illiteracy
- Research subjects are embarrassed to clarify and ask questions about the DNP project
- Worry and/or concern that failing to participate in the DNP project will impact their healthcare and/or treatment plan
- Fear of negative consequences for withdrawing early from a DNP project
- Vulnerable populations are diverse; so check with your DNP project mentor/chair before selecting a DNP project group

DNP, doctor of nursing practice.

SUBMISSION OF AN IRB APPLICATION

The first step in completing and submitting the IRB application is to carefully read and review each and every component of the IRB process available on the institution's website. For example, if the DNP students are submitting their DNP project to their workplace for IRB approval, the guidelines for the workplace must be followed. If the DNP students have no IRB committee in their workplace, they need to prepare their IRB application according to their university policies. When preparing their IRB packet, DNP students should allow time to complete a checklist so that all forms and guidelines are completed. Box 3.5 provides the DNP students with key advice as to how to prepare their IRB packet.

IRB APPROVAL AND IMPLEMENTATION OF THE DNP PROJECT

The IRB process may take various lengths of time depending on how complicated the project may be. For example, an expedited review may take only a short time over a few weeks (usually 2 or 3 weeks), whereas a full review may take several weeks to months. DNP students will need to become familiar with the IRB sites and information regarding submission and meeting dates and for the various types of IRB reviews. The DNP project timeline should include IRB approval since DNP students

BOX 3.5 Advice for DNP Students When Preparing the IRB Application

---

- Take time to carefully review and read all the details on the IRB application process.
- Use consistent terms from beginning to end in the IRB application.
- Write in a logical and sequential manner taking the IRB committee member from one idea to the next in a clear and succinct manner.
- Assume the IRB committee members know nothing about the content or topic of your DNP project.
- Describe the DNP project so that the IRB committee does not have to ask one question about what you are meaning or describing in your application.
- Be concise and succinct including only necessary information for each section of the IRB documents and the IRB application.
- Spell-check your work before submitting.
- Have a colleague or friend read and comment on your IRB application before submitting to your DNP faculty or project chair.
- Allow your DNP faculty or project chair time to thoroughly review and comment with feedback on your IRB application before submitting.
- Organize and submit the IRB application so that you do not miss any documents.
- Be patient and allow several iterations in this process.
- Be certain to allow a bit of extra time to carry out and complete the DNP project, allowing for any unforeseen delays or setbacks of any kind. It is better to have more time than not enough time.

IRB, Institutional Review Board.

may not begin implementation of their DNP project until they have received written IRB approval.

DNP students should work closely with the IRB and the DNP faculty mentor or chair for guidance and support to have their IRB application in proper order with all requisite documents and forms to make the IRB review process successful on the first attempt. If there are any changes to the DNP project once the DNP student has received final IRB approval, these changes must be submitted to the IRB in the form of an amended DNP application. Each IRB will have explicit details about how and what to submit if an amendment is needed. Again, the DNP project cannot be conducted until the IRB provides written approval for any amendment to the DNP project.

COMPLETION OF THE DNP PROJECT AND FINAL IRB REPORTS

Once the DNP project is concluded, there are still summary IRB forms to be completed. For example, there are IRB final reports to conclude and/or summarize the DNP project according to the specific IRB protocols. The DNP student is responsible for all of the IRB forms required by the IRB to close the project. Once the IRB closes the DNP project, the DNP student should file the forms according to the university or college guidelines. All final IRB reports are the DNP student's responsibility to complete prior to graduation.

SUMMARY

This chapter has focused on the need for the IRB process and the DNP project. An overview of the history of the IRB, strategies and considerations for writing an IRB application specific to the organization granting IRB approval, and types of IRB reviews were discussed. Throughout this chapter, there was specific emphasis on IRB issues related to the approval and protection of human subjects, particularly vulnerable populations involved in DNP projects. Additional content included topics about understanding the purpose and focus of the IRB related to the DNP project. Other areas included the definition of human subjects, creating a realistic timeline for the IRB application, understanding the IRB submission and approval process, understanding the need for following and adhering to the approved IRB protocol, and informed consent. Emphasis was provided about the need to understand one's responsibility in the completion of all IRB forms from the beginning of the project until the end of the project.

APPLICATION EXERCISES: PREPARING AND SUBMITTING AN IRB APPLICATION FOR A DNP PROJECT

Introduction

IRB approval for the DNP project can be labor-intensive and time-consuming. Many DNP students have never completed an IRB application or experienced the process. Lack of knowledge, skills, and preparatory work for the IRB application or not allowing adequate time for submission of the IRB application are issues that involve persistence. For example, the IRB application is a very technical document and the wording must be consistent with the IRB protocol language and include research terminology consistently from the beginning to the end of the document. Failure to prepare a well-developed IRB application according to the specific protocol requirements may result in the IRB application being returned for revision. Getting an IRB application returned for revision results in loss of time, which can extend from hours to weeks and sometimes months depending on the IRB review cycle and meeting dates.

The DNP student has to work with a variety of key stakeholders and key players during the IRB application process as well with key IRB personnel and staff once the document is submitted. It is advisable that the DNP student work in close collaboration with his or her DNP project faculty since faculty are familiar with the IRB process. Additionally, the DNP project faculty will have to sign the IRB application form and provide editorial assistance to the student. The DNP student should become intimately familiar with the IRB process and accompanying timelines during the DNP project planning and development phase. This will allow ample time to submit the appropriate IRB application and assist the student in keeping on a designated timeline.

Case Presentation

Sally Jones is in the final year of her DNP program. The DNP committee has approved Sally's DNP project proposal. The healthcare organization in which Sally works and will complete her DNP project does not have an IRB committee. Sally is not sure what to do in terms of the IRB process at this point. Sally knows she has extreme time limitations and a short window of opportunity in which to prepare her IRB application (see Appendix 3.1) and get approval (see Appendices 3.2 and 3.3) in order to complete her DNP project and graduate on time.

Application Exercise Questions

1. What are the first steps Sally should take to have a solid plan for preparing and submitting her IRB application?
2. Why must Sally's DNP project go through the IRB process?
3. What is the purpose of the IRB?
4. Where will Sally locate information on the IRB process that she should follow?

5. Who are the key stakeholders and key players Sally will be collaborating with during the IRB application process?
6. What communication strategies should Sally consider when completing the IRB application if she has questions at any time during the process?
7. What problem-solving strategies should Sally use if she is confused or unclear at any time during the IRB application process?
8. Discuss four common barriers/challenges Sally may experience in the IRB application process.
9. Identify four positive coping strategies Sally can apply as needed while completing the IRB application and process.
10. Examine how creating a Gantt chart is useful for having a successful experience completing the IRB process for one's DNP project.

REFERENCES

Al-Sheyab, N. A., Alomari, M. A., Khabour, O. F., Shattnawi, K. K., & Alzoubi, K. H. (2019). Assent and consent in pediatric and adolescent research: School children's perspectives. *Adolescent Health and Medical Therapy, 11*(10), 7–14. doi:10.2147/AHMT.S185553

Baines, P. (2015). Let's be clear about children and young people. *American Journal of Bioethics, 15*(11), 16–17. doi:10.1080/15265161.2015.1088983

Biros, M. (2018). Capacity, vulnerability, and informed consent for research. *Journal of Law, Medicine & Ethics, 46*(1), 72–78. doi:10.1177/1073110518766021

The Collaborative Institutional Training Initiative. (2018). Retrieved from https://about.citiprogram.org/en/homepage

Ingham-Broomfield, R. (2017). A nurse's guide to ethical considerations and the process for ethical approval of nursing research. *Australian Journal of Advanced Nursing, 35*(1), 40–47.

National Commission for the Protection of Human Subjects of Biomedical and Behavior Research. (1979). *The Belmont Report.* Retrieved from https://www.hhs.gov/ohrp/regulations-and-policy/belmont-report/read-the-belmont-report/index.html

Perrin, K. (2014). *Planning and evaluation for public health.* Burlington, MA: Jones & Bartlett.

U.S. Department of Health and Human Services, Office of Human Research Subjects Protection. (2018). *45 CFR 46.102(F) 2018 Requirements, PART 46—PROTECTION OF HUMAN SUBJECTS Subpart A—Basic HHS Policy for Protection of Human Research Subjects.* Retrieved from https://www.hhs.gov/ohrp/regulations-and-policy/regulations/45-cfr-46/index.html

APPENDIX 3.1: EXAMPLE OF A DNP IRB SUBMISSION

(Format dependent on the affiliated university/college)

Submit (by mail or email) the completed form to: IRB, University or College

Office of IRB Review

Name of University/College

PROPOSAL TITLE: Effects of an Evidence-Based Educational Intervention to Increase Nurse Educators Physical Activity at Work and at Home

INVESTIGATOR(S): *Insert DNP student name and faculty member name*

DEPARTMENT: *Add name of department or school*

FACULTY _ STUDENT_____

ADDRESS:

TELEPHONE NUMBER: *List direct phone number for principal investigator (DNP student)*

FACULTY ADVISOR (*if student*): _____

TYPE OF REVIEW REQUESTED: Full_____ Expedited__X___

IF EXPEDITED REVIEW, indicate the section(s) from the IRB guide under which this proposal qualifies for expedited review:

FULL OR EXPEDITED REVIEW" Check the appropriate response:

____YES ____NO

The protocol involves human subjects who will receive drugs.

____YES____NO

The protocol involves human subjects who will receive or be exposed to radioactive materials.

____YES ____NO

The protocol involves human subjects and will take place in an outside facility. ___YES__NO.

The protocol involves human subjects who are: ___minors (under age 18), ___fetuses, ___pregnant women, ___prisoners, ___mentally retarded, ___mentally disabled.

The protocol is being submitted for ___ Federal funding, ___Other external funding.

Purpose of the Study

The purpose of this evidence-based practice (EBP) is to help nurse educators develop sustainable behavior change strategies to increase physical activity at work and at home. The PICOT statement for this Doctorate of Nursing Practice (DNP) EBP final project is "In a population of nurse educators over the age of 18 working in a large urban nursing education program (Population), how does an evidence-based educational intervention help nurse educators develop sustainable behavior change strategies to increase physical activity at work and at home (Intervention) as measured on pre- and posttest intervention scores on the Exercise Benefits–Barriers Scale (EBBS) (Outcome) by the same group of nurse educators (Control) over 8 weeks (Time)."

Nurse educators are a population who may not get as much planned exercise and activity at work and at home as they need, resulting in elevated body mass index (BMI). A high BMI greater than 30 predisposes nurse educators to chronic health issues like chronic disease and illnesses like heart disease and stroke, respiratory problems, and muscle and joint problems. The purpose of this DNP EBP final project is to identify and assess perceived benefits and barriers of nurse educators to create a sustainable behavior change, promoting increased physical activity at work and at home to keep the BMI within normal range.

The Problem

Many nurse educators are working in sedentary occupational roles presently. Nurses who complete fewer than 5,000 steps per day are considered to have sedentary occupational sitting time (Munir, et al., 2015). Nurses completing fewer than 5,000 steps per day are at risk for preventable chronic disease and higher risk for increased mortality and morbidity from being overweight. Overweight nurses also have a difficult time serving as role models for their patients with regard to living active lifestyles and maintaining a healthy body weight (McEachan, Conner, Taylor, & Lawton, 2011). Overweight nurses are also more likely to experience poor health and chronic disease resulting in higher absence from work, exit early from the nursing workforce, or take early retirement (Parry & Straker, 2013).

Being overweight and particularly being obese substantially increases one's risk of morbidity and mortality from hypertension, dyslipidemia, depression, type 2 diabetes, coronary heart disease, stroke, gallbladder disease, osteoarthritis, sleep apnea and respiratory problems, and endometrial, breast, prostate, and colon cancers (Shields, Carroll, & Ogden, 2011). Excess body weight is associated with all cases of mortality (Shields et al., 2011).

Nurses serve as role models for patients and populations in many diverse healthcare settings. It is relevant for nurses to protect their health status with physical activity to maintain a normal BMI. Nurses, particularly nurse educators, cannot serve as role models to the patients/populations they serve unless they personally embrace and emulate the health status they are trying to impart to patients/populations. For example, it is a challenge to talk with patients or populations about weight control and healthy BMI if the nurse is overweight. There is also an imperative for nurses working in sedentary roles in the workplace with respect to the nursing shortage. Nurse educators are a population of nurses who work in sedentary roles in the workplace. As more and more nurse clinicians and nurse educators assume sedentary occupational roles, the issues with obesity and limited physical activity as health risks will continue to increase, leading to more chronic disease states that might have been prevented.

Project Outcomes

Two of the most important aspects of an evidence-based project is to have a clear purpose and focused outcomes in order to choose a valid and reliable measurement instrument to help achieve project goals (Newhouse, 2006, p. 110). It is relevant and essential for nurses to focus on outcome measures to improve specific interventions and provide a "road map" for future generations (Whitman, 2004, p. 293). The five specific project outcomes for this DNP EBP final project are to:

1. Examine general levels of perceived benefits and barriers to exercise of nurse educators in a large urban college of nursing regarding benefits and barriers to exercise (EBBS) pre- and post-evidence-based educational intervention
2. Identify what nonexercising nurse educators perceived to be the biggest benefits of exercise

3. Identify and assess what nonexercising nurse educators perceived to be the biggest barriers to exercise
4. Identify how nonexercising nurse educators' perceptions of benefits from exercise are related to their perceptions of barriers to exercise
5. Examine the impact (effect) of the evidence-based educational intervention on nurse educators' pre- and postintervention scores on the EBBS

Study Population

The PICOT statement for this DNP EBP final project is "In a population of nurse educators over the age of 18 working in a large urban nursing education program (Population), how does an evidence-based educational intervention help nurse educators develop sustainable behavior change strategies to increase physical activity at work and at home (Intervention) as measured on pre- and posttest intervention scores on the Exercise Benefits–Barriers Scale (EBBS) (Outcome) by the same group of nurse educators (Control) over 8 weeks (Time)."

Methods and Procedures

Research Design
The design for this DNP EBP final project is the pretest–posttest design. The population of nursing faculty will complete the EBBS consisting of 43 items and two qualitative questions at time 1. The evidence-based educational intervention to increase activity and decrease barriers to exercise and activity during the workday and at home will be administered via a web-based platform at the nurse educator's leisure; 4 to 6 weeks after the evidence-based educational intervention, the EBBS and qualitative questions will be readministered via Survey Monkey.

Mixed methods research is when the researcher uses both a qualitative phase and a quantitative phase in the research study. This DNP EBP final project includes mixed model research as a 43-item questionnaire, which will be uploaded into Survey Monkey and qualitative questions will be on the same questionnaire. The quantitative portion of the mixed methods design for this EBP project consists of administering the EBBS via Survey Monkey.

The qualitative portion of this mixed methods design for this EBP project consists of including open-ended qualitative questions at the end of the EBBS in Survey Monkey. The qualitative questions will be developed, allowing respondents to provide their individual responses related to exercise benefits and barriers in their workplace and at home.

How the EBBS Will Be Completed
The EBBS will be created in Survey Monkey or in Qualtrics by this DNP student. The nurse educators will receive an email asking them to participate in this DNP EBP final project. If the nurse educators choose to participate in this DNP EBP final project, their response will indicate they are giving informed consent. This will be thoroughly and carefully explained in the Research Consent Form. Once the DNP student receives the signed informed consent document, the nurse educator will be sent the link with a user ID and password to enter Survey Monkey to complete the initial preintervention EBBS survey.

Estimated Time Involved in Administration of the EBBS Through Survey Monkey
One of the authors of the EBBS will determine how long it will take nurse educators to complete the EBBS through Survey Monkey. It is anticipated completing the 43 items will take approximately 15 minutes.

Scoring of the EBBS and the Four Qualitative Questions
For purposes of this EBP project, the EBBS instrument will be scored as two separate scales. The advantage to scoring using two separate scales and scoring barriers and benefits to exercise separately is that the scores on the barrier scale items do not need to be reversed. It is this DNP student's thought that not having to reverse scores on the barrier scale will lessen the chance of data or statistical error. The other reason for computing a separate score for the EBBS benefits and barriers is to assist in identifying benefits and barriers to exercise for the nurse educators participating in this DNP EBP final project.

When the benefit scale is used separately, the score range is between 29 and 116. The higher the score, the more positively the individual perceives exercise. When the barrier scale is used separately, the score range is between 14 and 56. The higher the score on the barrier scale, the greater the perception of barriers to exercise. The higher the score, the more positively the individual perceives exercise.

Two qualitative questions are to be added to Survey Monkey to meet these DNP EBP project outcomes. The method of data analysis for the two qualitative questions is described and discussed in the data analysis section of this paper.

Sample

This DNP EBP final project focuses on an EBP intervention. PICOT questions on interventions focus on the intervention that most effectively leads to an outcome (Melynk & Fineout-Overholt, 2015, p. 28). For example, this specific DNP EBP final project focuses on the impact of an evidence-based educational intervention to help nurse educators develop and apply evidence-based strategies to increase their physical activity while at work and at home. The sample for this DNP EBP final project is one group of nurse educators for this project. The population of interest is nurse educators over the age of 18, teaching in a large, urban academic institution in Philadelphia, Pennsylvania.

A power analysis will be conducted to determine the sample size needed to avoid making a type II decision error. It is essential that an evidence-based project like this one has an adequate sample size (Melynk & Fineout-Overholt, 2015, p. 468). A type II error is failure to reject a null hypothesis when the null hypothesis is indeed false resulting in an incorrect decision (Gay & Airasian, 2003). The sample size needs to be large enough to be representative of the entire population to be able to generalize findings with a high degree of confidence. The principal investigator (PI) of this DNP EBP final project is currently working with a statistician to compute the power analysis for the sample size.

Sampling Plan

A purposive sampling plan is being used to recruit the population of nurse educators over the age of 18 working in a large urban nursing education program. Purposive sampling is a nonprobability sampling type and a nonrandom sampling technique utilized with quantitative research (Terry, 2015, p. 143). Random sampling would enhance the robustness of this DNP EBP final project; however, random sampling is not a feasible sampling plan, given the human and financial resource constraints involved with this DNP EBP final project.

A purposive sampling plan is being used to locate individuals who match the characteristics of the population of interest (Terry, 2015, p. 143). It is believed by the PI of this DNP EBP final project that this EBP project will collect exploratory data regarding nurse educators as a specific population. Purposive sampling is a pragmatic choice for this DNP EBP final project as the PI has access to a population of nurse educators to carry out the EBP project.

RISKS TO THE SUBJECT: __YES ___NO. If subjects will be at risk, assess the probability, severity, potential duration, and reversibility of each risk. Indicate protective measures to be utilized.

BENEFITS: ___YES ____NO. Describe any potential benefits to be gained by the subject as well as benefits that may accrue to society in general.

INFORMATION PURPOSELY WITHHELD: ____YES ___NO. State any information purposely withheld from the subject and justify this nondisclosure.

CONFIDENTIALITY/Protection of Human Subjects: Describe how confidentiality of data will be maintained.

Protection of Human Subjects

Upon receiving approval for this DNP EBP final project from the university, the PI will complete all of the necessary documents for submitting the proposal to the university's IRB for expedited review. The university's IRB application and review process takes approximately 4 to 6 weeks for an expedited review and decision. Once IRB approval is received through the university's IRB, an email will be sent to all full-time nurse educators age 18 and older in the college of nursing inviting them to participate in this DNP EBP final project. Informed consent will be voluntary completion of the initial Survey Monkey inviting nurse educators to participate in the study describing the benefits and barriers about exercise at work and at home. The response of the nurse educators to participate in the EBP final project would be an intent to participate. The nurse educators will be informed they can stop participation from the DNP EBP final project at any time. The email will provide a detailed explanation and overview of this DNP EBP final project for potential participants. If the nurse educator chooses to participate in the project as a result of this initial Survey Monkey response, this will signify informed consent.

REFERENCES

Gay, L. R., & Airasian, P. (2003). *Educational research: Competencies for analysis and applications* (7th ed.). Upper Saddle River, NJ: Prentice-Hall.

McEachan, C. R., Conner, M., Taylor, N. J., & Lawton, R. J. (2011). Prospective prediction of health-related behaviors with the Theory of Planned Behavior: A meta-analysis. *Health Psychology Review, 5*(2), 97–144. doi:10.1080/17437199.2010.521684

Melynk, B. M., & Fineout-Overholt, E. (2015). *Evidence-based practice in nursing and healthcare: A guide to best practice* (3rd ed). Philadelphia, PA: Wolters Kluwer.

Munir, F., Houdmont, J., Clemes, S., Wilson, K., Kerr, R., & Addley, K. (2015). Work engagement and its association with occupational sitting time: Results from the Stormont Study. *BMC Public Health, 15*(3), 1427–1439. doi:10.1186/s12889-015-1427-9

Newhouse, R. P. (2006). Selecting measures for safety and quality improvement initiatives. *Journal of Nursing Administration, 36*(3), 109–113. doi:10.1097/00005110-200603000-00002

Parry, S., & Straker, L. (2013). The contribution of office work to sedentary behavior associated risk. *BMC Public Health, 13*(1), 1–10. doi:10.1186/1471-2458-13-296

Shields, M., Carroll, M. D., & Ogden, C. L. (2011). Adult obesity prevalence in Canada and the United States. *Advanced Nutrition, 2,* 368–369. doi:10.3945/an.111.000497

Terry, A. J. (2015). *Clinical research for the doctor of nursing practice* (2nd ed.). Burlington, MA: Jones & Bartlett.

Whitman, G. (2004). Nursing sensitive outcomes in cardiac surgery patients. *Journal of Cardiovascular Nursing 195*(5), 293–298. doi:10.1097/00005082-200409000-00003

SIGNATURE OF PRINCIPAL INVESTIGATOR* _____

_____

DATE _____

POSITION_____

FACULTY MEMBER/SIGNATURE/POSITION

_____

ATTACHMENTS, for example

1. Informed Consent Form(s)
2. Detailed Research Protocol
3. Health Promotion Model—Instruments to Measure HPM Behavioral Determinants: Exercise Benefits/Barriers Scale (EBBS) (Adult Version)

_____

FOR IRB USE ONLY
ACTION TAKEN: _____

DATE: _____

SIGNATURE/IRB CHAIRPERSON:

_____

APPENDIX 3.2: EXAMPLE OF AN IRB COMMUNICATION GRANTING APPROVAL TO BEGIN

Dear Sally Jones,

Thank you for submitting your revised application entitled "Effects of an Evidence-Based Educational Intervention to Increase Nurse Educators Physical Activity at Work and at Home." The XYZ University IRB has reviewed your application. You have received IRB approval and may now begin your DNP project.

Please see the attached letter.

You may now begin data collection.

Please let the IRB know if there are any changes in your protocol or any developments that change in your original proposal as submitted.

Feel free to contact me at cyd@XXXuniversity.edu with any questions.

Best,

XYZ IRB Committee Member

Best,

XYZ IRB Committee Member

APPENDIX 3.3: EXAMPLE OF AN IRB COMMUNICATION REQUESTING ADDITIONAL CLARIFICATION

Dear Sally Jones,

Thank you for submitting your revised application entitled "Effects of an Evidence-Based Educational Intervention to Increase Nurse Educators Physical Activity at Work and at Home." The XYZ University IRB has reviewed the revised application. Thank you for addressing our concerns related to confidentiality of participants. We have a couple of additional minor follow-up clarifications we would like addressed before processing your approval letter. Please see the attached letter.

Please submit a revision, highlighting the changes. Do not begin data collection until you have received final approval.

Feel free to contact me at cyd@XXXuniversity.edu with any questions.

II | DATA

4 DATA COLLECTION, MANAGEMENT, ENTRY, AND ANALYSIS

MAHER M. EL-MASRI | FABRICE IMMANUEL MOWBRAY

INTRODUCTION

The goal of the DNP project is to answer clinical questions by completing a systematic approach to the collection of clinical data, management, entry, and analysis. The principles associated with these concepts are an important step in the success and completion of the DNP project. As part of the DNP Essentials, it is important to present clinical evidence by evaluating data associated with the quality of patient care and provide the leadership necessary to implement clinical changes. Thus, the DNP project should demonstrate an understanding of how to use clinical data and provide scientific evidence that will impact on clinical practice. This chapter is divided into sections with subheadings to assist in the understanding of the use of data. The first section focuses on understanding the "five Ws" (who, what, where, when, and why) necessary for conducting clinical studies as well as on understanding the sample size. We then include a discussion about the different types of data collection methods such as self-report, observational, and biophysiological. The next section focuses on the different approaches to data entry and the importance of accurately coding the data for computer analysis. Finally, we include a general approach of the use of statistics for quantitative and qualitative data analysis. Examples of how to make the right choice about the type of data collection methods, how to enter the data accurately, and understand the importance of data analysis are presented.

TANDING DATA

ıe measurable objective and subjective behaviors, characteristics, or observations found in our surrounding environment. When sought for research purposes, data are gathered and organized in a systematic fashion to help us better understand relationships and outcomes of interest, which is referred to as data collection (Grove, Burns, & Gray, 2013). Depending on the research question, data can be quantitative or qualitative in nature. Qualitative data often involve narrative description of conversations or behaviors as they take place in their natural setting, whereas quantitative data involve presentation of information in numeric form (Polit & Beck, 2010). Although research studies often elicit either quantitative or qualitative data, mixed methods research elicits a combination of quantitative and qualitative data to provide the most insight about a phenomenon of interest (Creswell, 2014). Regardless of the type of data, the aim of the data collection process is to ensure that complete and accurate data are gathered to provide for credible and replicable analysis. Accuracy of data collection starts with a good understanding of the conceptual and operational definitions of all the study variables. A conceptual definition of a variable provides a theoretical meaning of the variable, whereas the operational definition refers to the measurement of the variable in a study (Grove et al., 2013).

Sources of data in nursing and healthcare research are either primary or secondary in nature. Primary data are information that is directly elicited from research participants for the purpose of investigating a specific research question (Louiselle, Profetto-McGrath, Polit, & Beck, 2007). Examples of primary data include, but are not limited to, patient interviews, self-report surveys, and real-time observations. Secondary data refer to existing data records that are initially collected for purposes other than those of the proposed research and are repurposed to answer new research questions (Louiselle et al., 2007). Examples of secondary data include administrative databases, existing research databases, medical records, and death certificates. Whenever feasible, it is recommended that primary data be used to ensure that all required data are collected and that information bias (errors in data measurement) is minimized. However, eliciting primary data may be unfeasible or resource-intensive such as in the study of rare disease conditions or when the research requires a large sample size. In these cases, the use of secondary data may be the more pragmatic option.

Data Collection

Data collection procedures are both an intricate and essential step in the research process. Errors in data collection result in distortion of our understanding of reality and findings that may not be replicable in future research (Kupzyk & Cohen, 2015). The "five Ws" (who, what, where, when, and why) is an approach that we recommend to be used by researchers to maximize the accuracy of the data collection process.

Who are the data intended for? When collecting data, we need to contemplate "who" we would like our data to be generalizable to? The answer to this question should be formulated when establishing the research eligibility criteria—the attributes and characteristics that must be met for an individual to be included in the study (Guyatt, Drummond, Meade, & Cook, 2015). Keep in mind however, that while too strict eligibility criteria limit the generalizability of your findings, a broad eligibility increases error due to increased heterogeneity among participants. Strict eligibility criteria mean the research findings can only be applied to the few unique individuals who meet the criteria. On the other hand, ambiguous or broad eligibility criteria may blur the target populations. Thus, it is important to ensure that eligibility criteria be thoughtfully formulated to properly identify and select participants who represent the target population.

What data are needed? The type of data to be collected is dependent on the research question(s) being investigated and the proposed data analysis plan. For example, a researcher who is interested in comparing the hospital length of stay between medical and surgical patients will have to determine the level of measurement of hospital length of stay (e.g., continuous, ordinal, or nominal) based on his or her plan for data analysis. In the case of research on archived data, the analysis plan will be formulated based on the nature and level of measurement of available data. For instance, if hospital length of stay in the previous example was measured on an ordinal scale—using range of stay days—data analysis will be conducted using Mann–Whitney U statistics. However, if length of stay was measured in actual days and the variable was deemed to have a normal distribution, independent samples *t*-test would be the most appropriate analysis. It is also important that data be collected on the most valid measure of a given variable. For example, a nurse researcher who examines the impact of a lifestyle intervention on long-term blood glucose control in patients with type 2 diabetes should use A1C, as opposed to fasting blood sugar, to measure blood glucose control. This is because A1C is the more valid and reliable long-term measure of blood glucose levels.

Where were the data collected? The setting in which the data are collected impacts the external validity of research. To illustrate this point, imagine that a researcher was interested in exploring the rate of mortality due to traumatic injury (e.g., motor vehicle accident, falls) in a local urban center. If the researcher gathers the data from a regional community hospital, one is likely to be misled since the rates of mortality are low in their region. This is because traumatic injuries are likely to be transported out of the region to trauma centers that are better equipped to handle such injuries. Similarly, if a researcher is interested in examining the severity of benign prostate hyperplasia (BPH) among local men, they are likely to be misled into concluding that most men with BPH have higher grades of the disease if they gather data from a local urological outpatient setting. This is because men are more likely to be referred to a urologist only when symptoms are present or bothersome. Both of the aforementioned scenarios demonstrate the importance of ensuring that the appropriate setting is accessed for data collection.

When were the data collected? The timing of data collection is another consideration that researchers should consider. Both the time in relation to present day and the time in relation to disease or symptom manifestation should be considered. To illustrate the importance of timing in relation to present time, assume that a researcher was interested in conducting a secondary data analysis but only has access to data that are three decades old. In this case, one should be cautious when drawing conclusions from the findings of such analysis because the healthcare system is very dynamic, and many practices could have changed in the course of three decades.

To illustrate the importance of timing in relation to disease or symptom manifestation, let us assume that a researcher was interested in examining if the current dosing regimen of Lasix (furosemide) in a long-term care facility was effective in managing fluid retention in patients with congestive heart failure. Ideally, morning simple weight is an objective measure of fluid retention. However, if the weight was obtained randomly throughout the day, varying weights would occur as a result of the amount of food and fluid intake by patients. We know that patients drink and eat throughout the day, and that they are likely to retain more fluid as the day progresses. Thus, to ensure consistency in weight measurement, it is important that weight be obtained for all patients at the same time and under similar conditions.

Why were the data collected? The reason for data collection is an important question to consider, especially when using archived data. Research data tend to be more detailed and accurate compared to administrative or clinical data. Despite the source and origin of the data, researchers need to ensure that they collect the right data so that they may properly answer the research question of interest. Another key consideration is to always attempt to collect data on patient important outcomes that are likely to change patient values and behaviors (Guyatt et al., 2015). For example, reporting to a patient that his or her hemoglobin A1C has dropped is unlikely to change dietary habits in patients with type 2 diabetes. However, putting the drop in A1C in a clinical context and reporting that such a drop will be associated with a decrease in their microvascular complications (e.g., retinopathy and kidney disease) is an outcome that a patient is more likely to value.

Sample Size

Prior to data collection, it is imperative that the sample size for a study be empirically determined. Thus, sample size calculation should always be conducted to ensure that an adequate number of participants are recruited. Researchers can do these calculations either manually or they may use a computer program. A common and free resource used for computerized sample size calculation is G*power (Faul, Erdfelder, Buchner, & Lang, 2009). In order to conduct proper sample size calculation, one will need to determine if the calculation should be based on the assumption of a one- or two-tailed alpha. Typically, a two-tailed alpha is utilized, unless the researcher is interested in only testing a unilateral or directional hypothesis (Field & Miles, 2010). An alpha of 0.05 and a power of 80% is the common practice for sample size calculation in nursing so that type I and type II errors are balanced. However, researchers may always decrease the alpha or increase power estimates for more conservative sample size calculation. Effect size is another requirement of sample size calculation. Effect size is the quantitative magnitude of a relationship (e.g., odds ratio, relative risk, absolute risk reduction; Kelley & Preacher, 2012). It is recommended that it be estimated based on the existing literature. However, if estimates from the literature do not exist, a conservative but clinically significant estimate of the anticipated effect size is recommended. Overestimating the effect size is likely to result in type II error, while underestimation will increase sample size requirements and may prolong data collection beyond the capacity of the researcher.

Sample size calculation is not predetermined; rather, it is determined based on data saturation. That is, data collection continues until the recruitment of more participants no longer provides new information beyond what has already been generated. Thus, qualitative researchers usually propose a range of participants versus an exact number of participants.

ᴛA COLLECTION METHODS

Principles of Psychometric Measures

In general, psychometric measures focus on the development and validation of assessment tools that measure abstract variables. In order to measure a phenomenon of study, researchers need to quantify (assign a numeric value) to their observations and ensure that the numeric value accurately measures what they intend to measure. Variables can be defined as concrete such as height, weight, and blood pressure or abstract such as depression, anxiety, and quality of patient care. Psychometric research captures the degree to which an individual experiences a concept and is referred to as questionnaires, surveys, scales, inventories, or instruments.

The use of psychometric measures requires that the measure is providing accurate data associated with the concept or variable of study. For example, if one is trying to obtain a score related to depression, then it is important that there are data associated with the validity and reliability of the depression scale that is used. Reliability is defined as the extent to which a psychometric instrument yields an accurate score. Validity refers to which the instrument measures what it is intended to measure (El-Masri, 2016b).

A reliable instrument demonstrates internal consistency, stability, and equivalency. Internal consistency reflects attributes associated with the concept of study or how well the items work together. For example, if one is measuring depression, statements associated with sadness, activities of daily living, and cognitive functioning may be items that provide internal consistency among the items that make up the instrument.

The second component of reliability includes stability of the measure or the ability of the instrument to provide similar results when administered more than one time to the same group of respondents under the same condition. An example is the administration of a depression scale to the same group of patients during the same time under the same conditions. Stability is established by correlating the test and retest scores.

The third concept associated with reliability includes equivalency. Equivalency is the degree to which different forms of the same instrument yield similar results. Often, testing for equivalency is completed by a psychometrician, who develops an alternate form of the instrument and then asks a group of respondents to complete the alternate form within a few weeks from the original measure. It is the correlation between the results from the two forms that determines equivalency; the higher the correlation, the stronger the evidence of equivalency.

Validity of psychometric instruments indicates the appropriateness of the instrument as a measure of a concept and has two characteristics: translational and criterion validity. Translational validity is the extent to which the concept has been captured by the instrument. Face validity and content validity would be the most common way to test for translational validity. For example, the concept of depression would include the theoretical knowledge about the concept of depression. In order to establish content validity, a panel of experts may be used to review the concept being measured (depression), and they will confirm the factors associated with depression that are found in the literature as well as use their expertise to establish the attributes associated with depression.

Criterion validity refers to the degree to which the psychometric measure (depression) corresponds to one or more existing instruments that have been used to be valid measures. For example, use of Beck's Depression Inventory (BDI) scale and the Minnesota Multiphasic Personality Inventory (MMPI) to establish criterion validity about the concept of depression should provide similar results about the concept of depression.

It is important for a researcher to ensure that when using an established psychometric instrument that a thorough investigation has been completed to include a review of the literature associated with the concept of interest and data about the validity and reliability of the instrument. Therefore, it is best for the researcher to provide evidence from the literature about the use of the psychometric measure so that there are no concerns about the appropriateness of the measure or overall findings of the study.

Self-Report Methods

Self-report methods require that participants respond to a set of questions that elicit information about their personal attitudes, characteristics, behaviors, or circumstances (LoBiondo-Wood & Haber, 2010; Louiselle et al., 2007). Data using self-report measures can be obtained through direct interviews with participants, paper and pencil, or online. Interviews and focus groups are commonly used as qualitative data collection methods (Gill, Stewart, Treasure, & Chadwick, 2008), whereas surveys and questionnaires are more commonly used to obtain quantitative data. Self-reports are the most commonly utilized data collection method in nursing research and are often used to elicit information on outcomes that cannot be directly measured by biophysiological instruments (LoBiondo-Wood & Haber, 2010; Louiselle et al., 2007).

Self-report measures can be either descriptive or psychometric in nature. A descriptive survey is one in which each question elicits information on a stand-alone variable. Psychometric self-report measures, on the other hand, are those in which all questions or items are used as proxy measures of a single concept (El-Masri, 2016a). If a self-report measure is used for the latter purpose, it needs to include evidence of being both a valid and a reliable measure of the concept it is supposed to measure. Validity of a self-report measure refers to the extent to which it measures what it is supposed to measure (El-Masri, 2016b; Kimberlin & Winterstein, 2008). Reliability, on the other hand, refers to a measure's ability to accurately measure what it measures (El-Masri, 2016c; Grove et al., 2013).

A key limitation of self-report measures is that they are subjective, and it is therefore often difficult to ascertain if the respondent is telling the truth. This type of response bias is often driven by "social desirability," which reflects people's tendency to give socially acceptable answers even if those answers do not truly reflect how they experience the matter in question (Polit & Beck, 2010). Another limitation of self-report measures is that they are subject to misunderstanding by respondents, especially when they are poorly written or are written at a level that is higher than that of the participants.

Observational Methods

Observation is another data collection method often used to gather information on participants' conditions, communication, and environment (Polit & Beck, 2010). In observations, researchers collect data based on direct physical observations or through the use of prospectively documented data. An advantage of observations is that it tends to yield more accurate data as it is a more objective approach to data collection. It also tends to guarantee the temporal relationship between the exposure (i.e., independent variable) and the outcome of interest. It is important to keep in mind, however, that individuals tend to alter their normal behavior when they know that their behavior is being observed; this introduces a potential for bias that threatens the validity of observations.

Biophysiological Methods

Biophysiological measurement involves the use of equipment to determine the biological or physical status of a study participant (LoBiondo-Wood & Haber, 2010). Biophysiological measures are classified into either in vivo or in vitro measures (Louiselle et al., 2007). In vivo measure. performed directly on research participants. Examples of in vivo m sures include blood pressure, temperature, and pulse oximetry. On th other hand, in vitro measures use biophysiological material gathered from the participant that is then analyzed in a separate laboratory setting. Examples of this would be the growth of blood cultures and tissue biopsies (Louiselle et al., 2007). The advantage of using biophysiological measures is that the data collection methods are objective and precise as patients cannot distort these values intentionally as often found with self-report measures (LoBiondo-Wood & Haber, 2010). Furthermore, biophysiological measures are often plentiful and can often be found readily available in secondary data sources. When using biophysiological measures, it is important to ensure that they have sound sensitivity and specificity indices. Sensitivity of the measure refers to the proportion of cases that have the condition and properly identified as such by the measure. Specificity of the measure refers to the proportion of individuals who do not have the condition and are properly classified as such by the measure. While we strive to use measures that are both highly sensitive and specific, the trade-off between the sensitivity and specificity of a measure is often dependent on our intended purpose of use (i.e., ruling in versus ruling out a disease). If the goal is to rule in disease, one would be especially interested in using a sensitive measure. If the purpose was however to rule out disease, one would be more invested in using a specific measure.

CHOOSING A STATISTICAL METHOD

The use of statistical tests should be based on the type of study design. If one is using a quantitative design, then the use of descriptive, inferential, or hypothesis statistical testing would be appropriate. It is best to develop the statistical analysis prior to starting the study, at the stage of planning, and when the sample size is chosen. The statistical test chosen is dependent upon the research question that will be asked. Other determining factors are the type of data being analyzed, the number of groups or data sets involved, and the total number of participants.

For quantitative clinical studies, it is best to ask a set of questions associated with the use of numeric or categorical data. Questions associated with the differences between groups, variables used in the study, and types of data sets used will help to determine the best statistical method. Listed in the following are a set of generic research questions that may be helpful when determining the best statistical test to use (Nayak & Hazra, 2011)

- *Question 1: Is there a difference between groups that are unpaired?* Different statistical measures are required for numeric or categorical data. For numeric data, parametric tests are applied if there is a normal distribution; however, if the distribution is not normal, it is best to use nonparametric measures. When comparing more than two sets of numeric data, multiple group comparison is best.
- *Question 2: Is there a difference between groups that are paired?* Pairing refers to repeated measures on the same set of subjects. Pairing will occur if subject groups are different, but values in one group are linked or related to the other group (e.g., twin studies or parent–offspring studies). Multiple data set comparisons may need to be done through appropriate multiple group tests followed by post hoc tests.
- *Question 3: Is there any association between variables?* For numerical data, the statistical measures are testing for an association between two variables. These correlations express strength of the association as a correlation coefficient. An inverse correlation between two variables is depicted by a minus sign whereas a perfect correlation varies from 0 to 1. When two numeric variables are linearly related, then a linear regression model may be applied. For epidemiologic studies, an odds ratio and relative risk are used to express the association between categorical data.
- *Question 4: Is there agreement between data sets?* This comparison is between a standard screening or diagnostic test versus the availability of a "gold standard" or a new screening test or procedure. For example, scores from one data set may be compared with scores from a second data set, and it is the agreement between ratings of the scores given by different observers that would determine the difference between the two groups. Quantitative calculation of the correlation coefficient provides differences when comparing two data sets (Parikh, Hazra, Mukherjee, & Gogtay, 2010).

For qualitative studies, data analysis is determined by the qualitative method (grounded theory, phenomenological) chosen for the study. Qualitative data analysis involves the identification, examination, and interpretation of patterns and themes from textual data and determines how these patterns or themes help answer the research question. Qualitative data analysis refers to the processes and procedures used to analyze data and provides some explanation, understanding, or interpretation.

In general, qualitative analysis includes a series of steps v lyzing data:

1. Content analysis: This analyzes and interprets verbal data that can be analyzed descriptively.
2. Narrative analysis: This is analysis of text that may come from interview guides, surveys, written notes, or diaries. It often involves the development of stories or experiences of the people in the study.
3. Discourse analysis: This is concerned with the social context and how communication occurred. It focuses on the type of language used and how language from people expresses their everyday life experiences.
4. Grounded theory: This attempts to develop causal relationships about the way a phenomenon is presented, such as case studies or similar statements that are presented by the individuals in the study. Qualitative data analysis is likely to change as the study evolves or as the data emerge. This results in an ongoing, fluid, and cyclical process that happens throughout the data collection stage as the project carries over to the data entry and analysis stages.

It is important to note that qualitative data analysis is an ongoing, fluid, and cyclical process that happens throughout the data collection stage of the evaluation project and carries over to the data entry and analysis stages. Although the steps are somewhat sequential, they do not always (and sometimes should not) happen in isolation of each other. As the researcher moves between or within each qualitative analysis phase, it is important to always keep some guiding questions in mind that will reflect back on the study's purpose, research questions, and potential (Creswell, 2014).

DATA ENTRY

Quantitative Data Entry

Data entry is a bridging step between data collection and data analysis. Accurate data entry is essential to ensure that data analyses produce valid estimates of population parameters of interest. Data entry is, however, an error-prone task in which invalid entries are often not detected by statistical software or procedures, making it all so important to meticulously appraise and double-check data entry (Kupzyk & Cohen, 2015).

Normally, research data are collected on hard copies before they are transferred into electronic databases. This practice increases the chances of data entry error and makes the process of searching for data entry errors more tedious and time-consuming (Kupzyk & Cohen, 2015). With the mounting popularity of computer and smart device applications, there is a growing movement in the scientific community to directly collect and enter data into computer programs to decrease the risk of human error. Using computer applications also decreases the number of transfers of data and shortens the data collection time.

Prior to data entry and data analysis, data must be meticulously screened for errors (Grove et al., 2013). The data entry process should be systematic and uninterrupted to ensure that it is as error free as possible. It is recommended that data entry periods be limited to 2-hour segments to prevent fatigue-related errors (Grove et al., 2013). Make sure to back up data after each entry segment in an encrypted online or external storage apparatus to ensure no data are lost and to have data backed up in an encrypted external hard drive (Grove et al., 2013). Data coding is a common preliminary task of data entry that involves translating the entered data into an analyzable numeric form (Louiselle et al., 2007). For example, medical patients may be assigned a value of "0" while surgical patients may be assigned a value of "1".

Qualitative Data Entry

Data collection for qualitative research often occurs in real time, whether it is through field notes during an interview, observation, or examination of text or visual data. If data are recorded via an audio recorder, it needs to be transcribed—converted verbatim from spoken to written words to allow for a meaningful analysis (Sutton & Austin, 2015). Data entry for qualitative studies typically involves coding—a process of assigning and attributing terms to categories of data (text, visual, etc.; Creswell, 2014). Typically, codes are generated as more data are collected and analyzed. Creswell (2014) reports that coded data are typically organized into three categories: expected topics, unexpected topics, and topics that may provide conceptual interest to readers.

Qualitative data can be coded, entered, and analyzed either by hand or by computer programs such as "NVivo" and "ATLAS" (Creswell, 2014). Computerized data coding is gaining popularity due the tedious and time-consuming nature of manual approaches. It is important to note however that, unlike quantitative data analysis programs, computer programs do not actually analyze qualitative data. Instead, qualitative software is used to code and organize the data. Researchers are required to create, code, and organize the data, and search for both implicit and explicit themes (Wong, 2008).

QUANTITATIVE DATA ANALYSIS

Once data have been entered into a statistical software, they can be screened and managed in preparation for analysis. This is because raw data are rarely ready for analysis (Louiselle et al., 2007). Data screening is an extremely important step to ensure that all assumptions of planned analyses are met. When examining the data, we are searching for erroneous entries or violated assumptions that may require attention, with emphasis especially focused on, but not limited to, missing data (El-Masri, Hammad, & Fox-Wasylyshyn, 2005), the presence of outliers (Mobray, Fox-Wasylyshyn, & El-Masri, 2019), and normality (Tabachnick & Fidell, 2013).

After data screening and treatment for assumptions are completed, one can proceed to perform the planned data analysis. Descriptive statistics of the sample characteristics are often the first analyses conducted. In studies that entail group comparisons, it is important that such characteristics be compared across the groups as well. Next, the researcher begins to conduct bivariate analyses to provide a preliminary understanding of relationships between the study variables and the outcome of interest. Bivariate analyses, however, examine the relationship between only two variables, assuming that such a relationship is unique. This is however hardly the case, and, as a result, bivariate analyses should always be interpreted with caution and should rarely be used as the terminal analysis. This is because results from bivariate analyses are often confounded. More appropriately, adjusted multivariate analyses should be used to examine the association between an independent variable and the outcome variable while accounting for the confounding effect that other variables may have on this relationship.

The type of multivariate analysis depends on the level of measurement of the dependent variable and the nature of the research question being investigated. For instance, linear regression analysis is appropriate for the study of normally distributed continuous outcomes (e.g., hospital length of stay, time disease free), while logistic regression analysis is appropriate for binary outcomes. Ensuring appropriate assumptions of multivariate analyses (e.g., multivariate normality, and absence of multivariate outliers and multivariate collinearity) is vital to ensure that the findings of such analyses are valid (Tabachnick & Fidell, 2013). For instance, a unique requirement for multivariate regression is that all independent variables must be either continuous or dichotomous in

nature. As a result, all categorical variables with more than two categories and all ordinal variables that lack normal distribution shall be dum-
my-coded (i.e., transformed into dichotomous variables), whereby the
number of resulting dummies equals the number of orders/categories
in the original variable minus one. This may result because one category
will be used as a reference against which findings from each dummy will
be compared against. The selection of the reference category is usually
theoretical so that interpretation of the findings is possible. For example, when dummy-coding "ethnicity" in a country that is predominantly
White Caucasian, it is appropriate to choose "White Caucasian" as the
reference category. This is because White Caucasians are the majority,
and thus it is easier to compare other races to White Caucasians. Proper
reporting of the results is another important point. The results section should be succinct and specific to the outlined research questions.
Wandering away from the proposed data analysis plan casts doubt about
the rigor of the analyses and threatens the overall validity of the study.

It is also important to keep in mind that a statistically significant
finding does not always translate into a clinically significant one (El-Masri,
2016d). Thus, it is important to not be so focused on statistical significance
regardless of clinical significance. This is because, with a large sample, it
is possible to have a statistically significant finding even if the effect size
was very minute. For example, a study might suggest a statistically significant association between oral contraception and breast cancer (relative
risk: 1.04, 95% confidence interval: 1.02–1.1). However, the relative risk,
which indicates the effect size of this association, is very small suggesting that consumption of oral contraceptives increases the risk of breast
cancer by only 4%. The question one should ask: Is an increased risk of
4% large enough to warrant stopping the use of oral contraceptive pills?
The answer to this question is what determines one's conclusion as to
whether or not the study findings are clinically significant.

Data collection is an important step that directly impacts the internal validity of research. Regardless of the type of design (quantitative or
qualitative), data analysis should be conducted based on a well-articu-
lated data collection plan. Data collection tools and procedures must be
appropriate to elicit the outcomes desired. For any research study, it is
important that valid and reliable measures be used to quantify the concepts or outcomes of a study. Data entry provides the bridge between
data entry and data analysis. Errors can occur during this process; thus,
it is important to check and recheck data so that the validity of one's
research findings is not violated. Data analysis procedures should be
planned according to the proposed research questions. It is important
that statistical assumptions of all proposed data analyses are met to
maximize the validity of research findings.

QUALITATIVE ANALYSIS

Unlike quantitative analysis that involves the use of the examination of objective and quantifiable measures, qualitative analysis explores and interprets patterns and themes in written audio or visual data. Qualitative analysis is conducted to gain a deeper understanding of a phenomenon, rather than testing it (Guyatt et al., 2015). It is important to note that qualitative data is a dynamic and ongoing process that continues from data collection to final interpretation (Creswell, 2014). Initiating data analysis early is the key to assisting with pattern identification while progressing with data collection. Given its complex and dense nature, qualitative data analysis often involves data reduction (Creswell, 2014). Data reduction is the process of highlighting and keeping important data, and disregarding or deleting unnecessary or redundant data. Data reduction is a crucial process that guarantees the focus of the analysis on the research question so that we obtain an accurate understanding of the phenomenon of interest.

Qualitative data analysis can be organized in one of two approaches: content or thematic analysis. Content analysis involves coding and identifying the occurrence of an event in textual, audio, or visual data based on categories created prior to the analysis. Thematic analysis, however, involves identifying and interpreting patterns, and organizing them based on the research questions of interest. If numerous researchers are involved, it is recommended that investigator triangulation is conducted—a process where numerous researchers collect, analyze, and interpret the data to examine the similarity of organization and interpretation of data (Guyatt et al., 2015). Once data have been coded and organized, they are then examined for interrelating themes or descriptions (Creswell, 2014) and are displayed in a way that provides clarity or meaning to the data in hand. For example, in a phenomenological study that examines the experience of adapting a healthy lifestyle due to a recent diagnosis of diabetes, one could organize and display the data based on patient feelings, perspectives, and experiences. The final step of qualitative data analysis involves the identification and organization of the data for dissemination. Qualitative authors often utilize report excerpts from original transcripts or field notes to enrich the text and provide the reader with a vivid image of the interactions or experiences of participants (Guyatt et al., 2015).

SUMMARY

This chapter provided an understanding of how to use data when answering the five Ws (who, what, where, when, and why). A discussion associated with the use of psychometric tests, self-reports, and observational and biophysical methods has been presented. An understanding of the importance of determining sample size and use of various approaches to collecting data and entering data were presented. Presentation of how to choose a statistical method was provided. Finally, examples associated with qualitative versus quantitative data collection methods and analysis were discussed.

APPLICATION EXERCISES: PSYCHOMETRIC MEASURES, VALIDITY, AND RELIABILITY

Introduction

Psychometric measures focus on the development and validation of assessment tools to measure variables consistent with the field of research. This activity is based on an understanding of psychometric measures. For this learning activity, the Mini-Mental State Examination (MMSE) will be used as the exemplar. The MMSE is accessed online (www.oxfordmedicaleducation.com/geriatrics/mini-mental-state-examination-mmse).

Please download a copy for your continued work on this application exercise.

Validity is defined as the extent to which a psychometric instrument is measuring what it is intended to measure. Reliability is defined as the extent to which the instrument generates accurate scores.

Case Presentation

Mr. Jacobs, age 68, presented to the clinic because his wife insisted that he should be evaluated because he seemed to be having increased forgetfulness. Mr. Jacobs's wife was in the room with him and she stated the following: He was becoming more and more forgetful by citing examples like forgetting his keys to the car, where he parked the car, not knowing the names of his grandchildren, and often forgetting where his home was located. She further stated that he frequently would forget the day of the week or even where the bathroom was located in his house. Last, she states that he had not been seen by a healthcare provider since he retired 3 years ago. Terry Smith, the FNP provider, decided to separate Mr. and Mrs. Jacobs so that she could assess his mental and physical health.

When obtaining a history on Mr. Jacobs, she noted that his answers were inconsistent. For example, he could recall events related to his childhood but he had difficulty with knowing the day of the week, or current events such as "who" the president of the United States was or his wife's first name. Other mental health changes that Terry noted were that Mr. Jacobs had difficulty noting an object she would hold up and trying to count backward from 100.

Mr. Jacobs's physical examination was unremarkable. His physical neurological results were normal except for his orientation to time, place, and other cognitive functioning. As a result of the clinical history, Terry decided to complete an MMSE on Mr. Jacobs. After completion of the MMSE, Mr. Jacobs scored 23. As a result of the MMSE, Terry met with Mr. and Mrs. Jacobs and discussed the possibilities of the diagnosis of dementia or other possible diagnosis. Additionally, Terry ordered the following referrals: gerontologist appointment, neurologist review, general laboratory blood screening, and psychological review.

Application Exercise Questions

1. Is the MMSE an appropriate psychometric test to use in this clinical situation?
2. Provide clinical evidence to use the MMSE for this situation.
3. Has this clinical measure been used with past patient populations? Provide examples.
4. Discuss the reliability of the MMSE for clinical application.
5. How has the MMSE demonstrated validity as a clinically applicable test?
6. How is the MMSE scored?
7. How would you initially interpret Mr. Jacobs's MMSE score?
8. How does the MMSE assist nurse practitioners to clinically evaluate the mental health status of patients?
9. Would the MMSE be an appropriate screening tool for general annual physical and mental health exams?
10. Can a patient's MMSE score change from one appointment to the next?

Scoring of the MMSE

The MMSE is divided into two sections, the first of which requires vocal responses only and covers orientation, memory, and attention; the maximum score is 21. The second part tests ability to name, follow verbal and written commands, write a sentence spontaneously, and copy a complex polygon. Maximum total score is 30. (Folstein, Folstein, & McHugh, 1975, p. 197)

Applying Psychometric Measures

The use of any psychometric tool is dependent on the variables that need to be measured. Often clinicians need to quantify the observations that they make during a clinical event. Abstract variables such as mental health, depression, social isolation, or quality of life are difficult to capture and cannot be directly measured. Psychometric research tries to develop the metrics associated with the concept of interest and are referred to as inventories, surveys, or scales.

The importance of using the most accurate psychometric measure is dependent on the phenomenon under study. For example, the use of the MMSE was developed as a short, suitable clinical test for older adults with dementia, concentrating on the cognitive aspects of mental functioning. However, the MMSE cannot be used to diagnose dementia.

The MMSE is reliable and valid instrument to measure cognitive functioning, reports in the literature about its clinical effectiveness and has been supported in the literature about its clinical effectiveness (Robinson, Tang, & Taylor, 2015). The reliability pertains to whether or not the instrument is accurately measuring what it is supposed to measure, in this case, cognitive functioning experienced by patients. The validity of the instrument refers to the appropriateness of the instrument to measure the concept, in this example, "cognitive functioning."

Evidence-based clinical research reports have shown that the MMSE is a valid and reliable instrument that can be used on a variety of patient populations as well as on a variety of cultural groups. For example, Harrison et al. (2015) and Naqvi, Haider, Tomlinson, and Alibhai (2015) have shown that the MMSE was able to accurately predict that individuals who have low MMSE scores have a greater propensity toward being diagnosed with dementia. In fact, the *NICE Pathways Dementia Diagnosis and Assessment* (2016) has been used to demonstrate that when the MMSE is used as a screening tool for cognitive functioning, clinicians can determine changes in patients by tracking MMSE scores over time. Finally, the MMSE has been demonstrated to be culturally sensitive. Jae Baek, Kim, Park, and Kim (2016) showed that when the MMSE was used on groups of Korean patients, the instrument was sensitive enough for measuring cognitive functioning and that culture was not a significant factor.

Recommendations

The DNP project investigates clinical scholarship and contributes to the improvement of patient care. Clinical projects that require the use of a psychometric tool to measure the phenomenon under study are necessary to promote changes in the delivery of patient care. The importance of using a psychometrically sound instrument that has valid and reliable data, which demonstrates that the tool can measure what it is supposed to measure, assists the DNP student in the further development of DNP projects that can contribute to or change clinical practice models.

It is recommended that DNP graduate students systematically review the use of any psychometric tool that they are interested in using while completing their project. Use of the 10-item questions as displayed earlier could be one format that could be utilized to investigate the validity and reliability of the instrument. The development of logic questions as a way to evaluate the psychometric tool that will be utilized with the DNP project will provide a systematic way to integrate the concepts that will be measured. This methodology will assist the student in the understanding of the phenomenon (concept) under study as well as assist the student in the overall interpretation of the clinical results.

Answers for the logic questions for the use of the MMSE have been provided as an example to assist in the evaluation of an appropriate clinical psychometric instrument that could be used for clinical practice.

REFERENCES

Arevalo-Rodriguez, I., Smailagic, N., Roque, I. F. M., Ciapponi, A., Sanchez-Perez, E., Giannakou, A., . . . Cullum, S. (2015). Mini-Mental State Examination (MMSE) for the detection of Alzheimer's disease and other dementias in people with mild cognitive impairment (MCI). *Cochrane Database Systematic Review, (3)*, 1. doi:10.1002/14651858.CD010783.pub2

Creswell, J. W. (2014). *Research design: Qualitative, quantitative, and mixed-methods approaches.* Thousand Oaks, CA: Sage Publications, Inc.

El-Masri, M. M. (2016a). Introduction to psychometric measurement. *Canadian Nurse, 111*(3), 13.

El-Masri, M. M. (2016b). Validity of psychometric measurements. *Canadian Nurse, 112*(4), 12.

El-Masri, M. M. (2016c). Reliability of psychometric measurements. *Canadian Nurse, 112*(5), 11.

El-Masri, M. M. (2016d). Focus point: Statistical versus clinical significance. *Canadian Journal of Nursing Research, 48*, 31–32. doi:10.1177/0844562116677895

El-Masri, M. M., Hammad, T. A., & Fox-Wasylyshyn, S. M. (2005). Predicting nosocomial bloodstream infections using surrogate markers of injury severity: Clinical and methodological perspectives. *Nursing Research, 54*(4), 273–279.

Faul, F., Erdfelder, E., Buchner, A., & Lang, A.-G. (2009). Statistical power analyses using G*Power 3.1: Tests for correlation and regression analyses. *Behaviour Research Methods, 41*, 1149–1160. doi:10.3758/BRM.41.4.1149

Field, A. P., & Miles, J. (2010). *Discovering statistics using SAS (and sex and drugs and rock 'n roll).* Thousand Oaks, CA: Sage Publications, Inc.

Folstein, M., Folstein, S., & McHugh P. (1975). "Mini-Mental State": A practical method for grading the cognitive state of patients for the clinician. *Journal of Psychiatric Research, 12*, 189–198. doi:10.1016/0022-3956(75)90026-6

Gill, P., Stewart, K., Treasure, E., & Chadwick, B. (2008). Methods of data collection in qualitative research: Interviews and focus groups. *British Dental Journal, 204*(6), 291. doi:10.1038/bdj.2008.192

Grove, S. K., Burns, N., & Gray, J. (2013). *The practice of nursing research: Appraisal, synthesis, and generation of evidence.* St. Louis, MO: Elsevier Health Sciences.

Guyatt, G., Drummond, R., Meade, M. O., & Cook, D. J. (2015). *User's guides to the medical literature: A manual for evidence-based clinical practice.* New York, NY: McGraw-Hill Education.

Harrison, J. K., Fearon, P., Noel-Storr, A. H., McShane, R., Stott, D. J., & Quinn, T. J. (2015). Informant Questionnaire on Cognitive Decline in the Elderly (IQCODE) for the diagnosis of dementia within a secondary care setting. *Cochrane Database Systematic Review, 3*, 1. doi:10.1002/14651858 .CD010772.pub2

Jae Baek, M., Kim, K., Park, Y., & Kim, S. (2016). The validity and reliability of the Mini-Mental State Examination-2 for detecting mild cognitive impairment and Alzheimer's disease in a Korean population. *PLoS One, 11*(9). doi:10.1371/journal.pone.0163792

Kelley, K., & Preacher, K. J. (2012). On effect size. *Psychological Methods, 17*(2), 137–152. doi:10.1037/a0028086

Kimberlin, C. L., & Winterstein, A. G. (2008). Validity and reliability of measurement instruments used in research. *American Journal of Health-System Pharmacy, 65*(23), 2276–2284. doi:10.2146/ajhp070364

Kupzyk, K. A., & Cohen, M. Z. (2015). Data validation and other strategies for data entry. *Western Journal of Nursing Research, 37*(4), 546–556. doi:10.1177/0193945914532550

LoBiondo-Wood, G., & Haber, J. (2010). *Nursing research: Methods of critical appraisal for evidence-based practice.* St. Louis, MO: Mosby Elsevier.

Louiselle, C. G., Profetto-McGrath, J., Polit, D. F., & Beck, C. T. (2007). *Canadian essentials of nursing research* (2nd ed.). Philadelphia, PA: Lippincott Williams & Wilkins.

Mobray, F. I., Fox-Wasylyshyn, S. M., & El-Masri, M. M. (2019). Univariate Outliers: A conceptual overview for the nurse researcher. *Canadian Journal of Nursing Research, 51*(1), 31–37.

Naqvi, R. M., Haider, S., Tomlinson, G., & Alibhai, S. (2015). Cognitive assessments in multicultural populations using the Rowland Universal Dementia Assessment Scale: A systematic review and meta-analysis. *Canadian Medical Association Journal, 187*(5), E169–E175. doi:10.1503/cmaj.140802

Nayak, B., & Hazra, A. (2011). How to choose the right statistical test? *Indian Journal of Ophthalmology, 59*(2), 85–86. doi:10.4103/0301-4738.77005

NICE Pathways. (2016). *Dementia diagnosis and assessment* (p. 10). Retrieved from https://www.nice.org.uk/about/what-we-do/our-programmes/about-nice-pathways

Parikh, M., Hazra, A., Mukherjee, J., & Gogtay, N. (2010). Research methodology simplified: Every clinician a researcher. New Delhi, India: Jaypee Brothers, Medical Publishers Pvt. Limited.

Robinson, L., Tang, E., & Taylor, J. P. (2015). Dementia: Timely diagnosis and early intervention. *BMJ, 350*, 1–6. doi:10.1136/bmj.h3029

Sutton, J., & Austin, Z. (2015). Qualitative research: Data collection, analysis, and management. *The Canadian Journal of Hospital Pharmacy, 68*(3), 226. doi:10.4212/cjhp.v68i3.1456

Tabachnick, B. G., & Fidell, L. S. (2013). *Using multivariate statistics* (6th ed.). Boston, MA: Pearson.

Wong, L. P. (2008). Data analysis in qualitative research: A brief guide to using NVivo. *Malaysian Family Physician: The Official Journal of the Academy of Family Physicians of Malaysia, 3*(1), 14.

III

THE CLINICAL STAFF AND INTERPROFESSIONAL COLLABORATION

5 DEFINING CLINICAL STAFF AND ROLES AND RESPONSIBILITIES

DENISE M. KORNIEWICZ

INTRODUCTION

Today, healthcare systems are constantly changing due to increased government regulations, consumer-driven healthcare, and the demand for new patient-centered technologies that require consistent monitoring for quality outcomes (Pittroff & Hendricks-Ferguson, 2018). As a result, clinical staff are inundated with learning new ways to provide safe patient care, decrease medication errors, and decrease hospital-acquired infection rates. Often, opportunities to conduct clinical research have become more complicated; thus, the DNP student may encounter some barriers when embarking on a DNP project. Regardless of the issues that a DNP student may encounter in the clinical setting, what is important is to be cognizant about the current trends in healthcare that may impact on the execution of the project.

Initially, the implementation of any evidence-based practice change in the current healthcare delivery system may be viewed as overwhelming for the DNP student. However, if the DNP project has a shared clinical purpose such as reducing the time it takes to provide patient care about a clinical problem, then the clinical staff would be more inclined to engage with the DNP student. Thus, a commitment of a shared purpose, openness, and sharing ideas, as well as building clinical relationships, provides a framework for successful implementation of the DNP project (Walsh et al., 2017).

There are several steps that need to be considered when developing the DNP project in the clinical environment. If the project requires that clinical staff be involved in the data collection process, then it is important to understand the various clinical team members, their role and responsibilities as well as the clinical environments in which the project will be completed. Often as a DNP student, one may or may not know the clinical facility when developing the clinical project. For example, one may need to rely on clinical staff to participate in certain procedures or conduct patient surveys. This chapter includes content to successfully complete a DNP project and provides: (a) assessment of the clinical environment for implementing the scholarly project; (b) identification of all the clinical staff that will be involved with the patient during the project period; (c) evaluation as to how to engage the staff in the project; (d) sustainment of the staff during the project period; and (e) debriefing the staff when the project is completed. Finally, this chapter provides the tools necessary for how the DNP student can be successful when implementing the project in any clinical environment.

ASSESSMENT OF THE CLINICAL ENVIRONMENT

There are a variety of healthcare environments ranging from inpatient units and specialty hospitals to community outpatient settings. Choosing the right clinical environment is dependent on the population of interest, the availability of patients, and the clinical question posed in the project proposal. The importance of understanding the clinical environment and the impact that the environment may have on the patient population provides insight as to how to conduct the DNP project within the structure and environment of the clinical setting.

Anaker, Heylighen, Nordin, and Elf (2017) found that the design of healthcare environments needed to be based on evidence. For example, being aware of the type of design quality in relation to the healthcare architecture helps when designing the physical healthcare environment. Furthermore, Anaker et al. (2017) provided three major concepts that promoted evidence-based healthcare designs: (a) environment sustainability, (b) social and cultural values, and (c) resilience of the building construction. Physical environments that are of high quality can be a therapeutic resource for promoting health and well-being (Gesler, Bell, Curtis, Hubbard, & Francis, 2004) as well as providing an approach for quality improvement for patient care (Freihoefer, Nyberg, & Vickery, 2013). The importance of understanding the interface of architectural evidence-based designs may impact the overall clinical research environment. Weller (2014) found that when the physical clinical environment was not upgraded to include changes in patient units, modernization of hospital work stations, or refitting of space for new hospital equipment, hospital personnel were less likely to support well-being and respect different social or cultural values. Furthermore, the lack of promoting an evidence-based approach to physical design in the clinical environment may indirectly affect communication and collaboration among healthcare personnel and impact on activities such as data collection, communication, or surveys during the time frame of the scholarly project.

There continues to be many challenges when conducting research in a clinical environment. Depending on the type of facility, the environment not only includes the patient but a cadre of healthcare providers such as nurses, nursing techs, laboratory techs, secretarial staff, physicians, physical therapists, and other specialists. The facility may be undergoing change and new roles and responsibilities may be redefined by management; thus the staff may be confused or unsure about the impact of these changes. Therefore, it is best to test the temperature of the clinical environment by assessing the following: (a) observation of the number of nurses per patient; (b) communication on the unit; (c) visibility of the charge nurse; (d) chaos versus calm environment; and (e) overall general cleanliness of the environment (Mourshed & Zhao, 2012).

Once an assessment has been completed on the clinical environment of choice, it would be best to develop an action plan and timeline to share with all of the clinical staff. Any negative observations or concerns should be discussed with the manager of the unit so that input can be obtained as to the best way to intervene during the project period. Based on suggestions from the unit manager(s), the action plan and timeline should be communicated to all clinical staff members so that they are aware of their contributions to the overall project.

IDENTIFICATION OF CLINICAL STAFF

During the assessment of the clinical unit, it is important to obtain data about the number and type of staff that are available daily as well as the type of staff that intermittently interact with the patient. Examples include but are not only limited to nursing staff but may also include a variety of other healthcare professionals who communicate or provide patient care. Identification of their roles and responsibilities would need to be documented so that it is representative of the healthcare workforce that was included during the scholarly clinical project period. Table 5.1 provides an example of how to present the role of the healthcare workforce that may be available during each phase of the clinical scholarly project.

TABLE 5.1 Identification, Definition of Clinical Staff, Number, and Role Responsibilities

Name of Clinical staff	Definition	Number per Shift	Role Responsibilities
RN	• Licensed healthcare professional who provides personal care to patients, administers medications, ensures overall quality of patient care	3	• Charge nurse of unit or primary care nurse over an assigned number of patients • Supervises ancillary help (LPN activities, nursing techs) • Oversees all patient care activities provided by licensed and unlicensed healthcare personnel
LPN	• Licensed healthcare professional who works under the direction of an RN • Provides patient care activities including the administration of oral medications • Responsible for providing patient care procedures consistent with patient care needs	1	• Provides patient care activities consistent with assignment from charge nurse • Accountable for oral medication distribution and timeliness of patient care • Follows up with charge nurse for any activities assigned
Patient care aide/technician	• Unlicensed personnel, varies by state, may need to be certified • Works under the direction of a licensed healthcare professional (LPN, RN, MD)	1–2	• Able to obtain patients' temperature, blood pressure, pulse, and respiration • Assists patients with basic tasks, such as bathing, dressing, and eating • Collects specimens for lab tests • Monitors patients and records data

(continued)

TABLE 5.1 Identification, Definition of Clinical Staff, Number, and Role Responsibilities (continued)

Name of Clinical staff	Definition	Number per Shift	Role Responsibilities
Laboratory technician	• Trained professionals responsible for performing complex tasks and procedures that are medical in nature	1	• Collects and analyzes body fluid and tissue samples for abnormalities • Operates laboratory equipment and other computerized tools in a laboratory setting
X-ray technician	• Certified and licensed health professional who performs imaging services that often lead to the timely identification of medical conditions, proper treatments, and even cures for a wide cross-section of patients	1	• Responsible for performing diagnostic medical imaging on patients • Responsible for adjusting and maintaining x-ray machine • Processes and stores x-ray film
Primary physician	• Licensed medical doctor who is responsible for the overall treatment of the patient	1	• Responsible for the diagnosis, treatment, and follow-up services needed by the patient
Specialty physician	• Licensed medical or surgical doctor • Board certified in area of specialty	1	• Responsible for completing consultation services ordered by the primary physician • Responsible for diagnosis, treatment, and follow-up services associated with their specialty

LPN, licensed practical nurse; RN, registered nurse.

ENGAGING CLINICAL STAFF

Engaging staff with the DNP project is essential for successful implementation and completion of the project. However, it is important to be aware of some of the issues that have been expressed by clinical staff members. For example, Finch, Cornwell, Nalder, and Ward (2015) noted that nursing staff expressed fear when asked to participate in quality assurance or research projects because they felt that they were inadequately trained or had insufficient skills for the research project. Others (Raymond, Profetto-McGrath, Myrick, & Strean, 2018) found that when staff were educated about the principles of basic research, then they were more likely to participate in evidence-based projects. Additionally, when the clinical agency is able to cultivate clinical staff within an environment of evidence-based practice and provide a clinical ladder consistent with compensation that is linked to performance goals, then a foundation for stronger research is built (Table 5.2).

DNP students should provide training sessions associated with the DNP clinical project to the staff to further an understanding about how their project will enhance clinical practice. Furthermore, it would guide the clinical staff in the understanding of their role and function when participating in a clinical project.

There are several other issues associated with engaging the clinical staff with the DNP scholarly project. MacPhee, Dahinten, and Havaei (2017) noted that the major issues that concerned the clinical staff included: (a) the amount of additional time that would be expected when providing patient care, (b) additional resources needed for compensation, and (c) a resource infrastructure to support any additional burden on managers or charge nurses to participate in the project. However, White (2012) found that if management provided support for a research-based clinical environment, then staff were more likely to engage in evidence-based clinical projects. Furthermore, if staff sought out opportunities to engage in quality assurance projects as an expectation for their annual review, then clinical staff would be more likely to participate in evidence-based clinical projects.

Finally, nurse staffing, patient acuity levels, and workload interruptions influence nurse outcomes (MacPhee et al., 2017) and indirectly is an issue when trying to engage clinical staff with the DNP projects. Unfortunately, job workload is based on the nurse's perceptions of the amount of work per day and nurse resources are based on the mental concentration to do the task (Holden et al., 2011). The cognitive demands expected of the staff nurse to participate in data collection, discussion groups or evaluation methods associated with a DNP project may be perceived as additional work or interruptions in routine patient care.

TABLE 5.2 The EBP Effectiveness Compendium

Selected Practices to Promote EBP Clinical Research

1 *Growing the EBP Base*	2 *Advancing EBP Development*	3 *Providing Ongoing EBP Support*	4 *Delivering EBP Performance Reviews*	5 *Aligning Compensation With Performance Goals*
1. Identified EBP clinicians	4. Nurse EBP leadership rotations	8. Integrated EBP clinical training teams	11. Successive internal reviews	14. EBP incentives
2. Leadership skills to evaluate EBP	5. Targeted training EBP	9. Strategic coaching EBP	12. Annual reviews EBP integration	15. Goal-driven compensation
3. EBP processes	6. Applied skills. EBP training	10. Provide EBP support positions	13. Comprehensive system reviews EBP	16. Achievement only—compensation
	7. Clinical leadership Training model			

EBP, evidence-based practice.

A few basic principles to use when engaging staff with a clinical project may include: (a) developing clinical relationships prior to the outset of the project; (b) making it easy for clinicians to participate; (c) identifying staff who can be champions of the project; (d) bringing together inter-disciplinary teams so that healthcare professionals can learn from each other; and (e) expressing gratitude to staff for their continued participation (Woolf, Zimmerman, Haley, & Krist, 2016). If it is at all possible, it is best for the DNP student to provide the personnel needed to complete data collection procedures that require additional time by the clinical staff. This will demonstrate the importance of the clinical project and validate the need for additional resources that may be needed by clinical staff when undertaking evidence-based clinical projects.

Once the DNP student has assessed the clinical environment, met the clinical staff, and has obtained the proper permission to conduct the clinical project, it would be important to plan out how to keep the clinical staff engaged in the project. One way to do this would be to set goals as to dates, times, and content that would be prepared to present to the clinical staff. Engaging staff in the process of the clinical project would ensure positive outcomes for data collection and/or the implementation of the clinical project (White, 2012). Table 5.3 presents an example of the content that could be covered weekly for a DNP project timeline.

SUSTAINING CLINICAL STAFF IN THE PROJECT

Depending on the educational institution with which the DNP student is affiliated, most DNP projects may take 8 to 14 weeks to complete. Therefore, being able to keep the clinical staff engaged in the project from beginning to end becomes necessary since the quality of the project is dependent on the successful involvement of the clinical staff. Each

TABLE 5.3 Example of Weekly Content for Clinical Staff Engagement in a DNP Project

Week	Suggested Content
1	Overview of project and timeline
2	Importance of data collection, accuracy, and review of data collection tools
3	Engaging clinical staff and project involvement
4	Discussion about the completion of project and appreciation of staff
5	Presentation of data, outcomes of study, and next steps

aspect of the clinical project will require precise data collection procedures to provide for the quality of the data retrieved, adherence to the inclusion and exclusion of patient data requirements, recruitment of the number of patients required for the project, and adherence to research protocols associated with the overall project.

Several authors (Bakken, Lantigua, Busacca, & Bigger, 2010) have suggested that clinical staff be provided with incentives to sustain their interest and participation throughout the project period. A few examples of incentives may include recognition as a collaborator in the overall research, continuing education credit, and already-paid coffee credit cards. Other incentives that have been found to assist in the sustainability of clinical staff in research projects may include: (a) organizational goals associated with promotion; (b) unit goals related to Magnet® status; (c) peer pressure due to team building; and (d) the ability to present at national research conferences (Hagan & Walden, 2017).

Regardless of the clinical project that has been undertaken, sustainability and continued interest to fulfill the project requirements is a key factor for the DNP student. For example, knowledge about how to communicate with the staff and maintain staff desire to work on the clinical project is of value (Scala, Price, & Day, 2016). In fact, Hagan and Walden (2017) noted that being available to interface with the staff directly during routine clinical shifts provided better project outcomes as measured in the number of patients recruited, number of completed data collection forms, and the accuracy of the data collected. Examples of how to sustain the staff's interest in the clinical project would include: (a) relevancy of the clinical topic; (b) quality improvement initiatives that are evidence-based; and (c) research activities that are realistic and achievable. One way to obtain information about how the clinical staff are responding to the DNP project would be to randomly meet with a small group of clinical staff members and complete a brief SWOT (strengths, weaknesses, opportunities, and threats) analysis within 3 to 4 weeks of the project. The SWOT analysis can be finished in a few minutes and can provide the DNP student with feedback so that corrections can be made in enough time to complete the desired outcomes of the project. By doing a SWOT analysis, it may open up other opportunities of communication or make changes that will allow for continued sustainability of the project. An example of questions that may be used while performing a SWOT analysis for sustainability can be found in Table 5.4.

Based on the communication with the clinical staff and use of a SWOT analysis, the DNP student would be able to tailor the DNP project to engage the staff and sustain them from beginning to end during the project period.

TABLE 5.4 Suggested Questions for a SWOT Analysis in the Clinical Environment

Analysis	Suggested Questions
S (Strengths)	• What advantages are there to conduct your clinical scholarly project at this institution? • What do you see as the strengths of this facility? • What do you see as the strengths of the clinical staff? • What factors can you list as important to your clinical scholarly project?
W (Weaknesses)	• What could you improve as a result of completing your clinical scholarly project with this healthcare facility? • What should you avoid when doing your clinical scholarly project? • What are the clinical staff likely to see as weaknesses? • What factors may impact on your clinical scholarly project?
O (Opportunities)	• What good opportunities can you suggest as a result of your clinical scholarly project? • What interesting trends in healthcare are you aware of that may impact on the results of your clinical scholarly project? • What changes in technology may enhance the impact of your scholarly project?
T (Threats)	• What obstacles do you face when implementing and completing your clinical scholarly project? • Are there competing issues that may impact your clinical scholarly project? If so, what can you do to enhance success of your project? • Are there quality standards or specifications about the clinical environment that are changing while you are completing your clinical scholarly project?

DEBRIEFING CLINICAL STAFF ABOUT THE PROJECT

Pittroff and Hendricks-Ferguson (2018) found that one reason the clinical staff are hesitant about working on clinical projects is because often they are not informed about the outcome of the project. Regardless of how large or small the clinical project was, the clinical staff needs to be informed about the outcome of the data obtained. Often, this step is forgotten or not implemented since it requires the DNP student to return and report back to the clinical staff after the analysis of data is completed. Clinical staff are interested in the findings of the project and like to know the results of the data. One way to provide feedback to the staff is to hold a debriefing session with them during shift change or at a time that is most convenient. The purpose of the debriefing is to provide information about the findings of the project. This can be completed via a roundtable discussion, lecture, or through a participatory discussion with the clinical staff.

Debriefings have been used to provide feedback to clinical teams and are used to discuss opportunities to improve individual, team, or system level issues (Cheng et al., 2017). Additionally, debriefings have been used to incorporate patient safety issues stemming from adverse clinical events. However, the same principles for a debriefing session about a DNP project can be used to discuss the findings or outcomes of the project. These principles may include issues associated with the following: (a) clear communication about the project; (b) understanding of the clinical role in the project; (c) maintenance of data collection tools; and (d) engagement of the staff. By using a format that is familiar to clinical staff, the DNP student may be more successful at engaging the staff when presenting the findings.

There are several key points associated with the findings of the DNP project that should be part of the debriefing session. Examples may include the use of reflective questions such as: (a) What went well? (b) What obstacles occurred during the project? (c) How could your role be enhanced during the project? (d) If the project were repeated, what would you suggest to improve the overall success of the project? (e) Why or why not would you participate in another clinical scholarly project? Use of reflective questioning has been successful as an active learning strategy to engage clinical staff members (Eppich & Cheng, 2015). Moreover, the educational research literature supports debriefing as an effective way to enhance adult learning and promote team performance (Hénard & Roseveare, 2012). Thus, understanding how to conduct a debriefing session as the facilitator of your project as well as knowing how to implement adult learning concepts provides a framework to conduct your debriefing session.

Discussion of the findings of one's study can be instrumental in making changes to clinical guidelines associated with the quality of patient care. Providing a debriefing session related to the DNP project will assist the staff in understanding the importance of their participation in evidence-based clinical projects. Suggestions from frontline clinical staff may provide insights about the findings from the DNP project and initiate further discussions that may improve one's interpretation of the results. The debriefing session about the final results presents direct communication about the DNP project findings and provides closure of the work with the clinical staff. This final step is necessary so that the clinical staff are acknowledged for their work on the DNP project and appreciated for their participation.

SUMMARY

This chapter provided examples as to how to be successful at assessing the clinical environment and identifying the appropriate clinical staff involved in the scholarly project. The importance of engaging and sustaining clinical staff with activities associated with the project was presented. The final section included a debriefing session that provided a framework for facilitating a debriefing session related to the findings of the project. The overall intent of this chapter was to assist the DNP student with successfully completing his or her project in any clinical setting.

REFERENCES

Anaker, A., Heylighen, A., Nordin, S., & Elf, M. (2017). Design quality in the context of healthcare environments: A scoping review. *HERD: Health Environments Research & Design Journal, 10*(4), 136–150. doi:10.1177/1937586716679404. Retrieved from http://www.creativecommons.org/licenses/by-nc/3.0

Bakken, S., Lantigua, R., Busacca, L., & Bigger, J. T. (2010). Barriers, enablers, and incentives for research participation: A report from the ambulatory care research network (ACRN). *The Journal of the American Board of Family Medicine, 22*(4), 436–445. doi:10.3122/jabfm.2009.04.090017

Cheng, A., Grant, V., Huffman, J., Burgess, G., Szyld, D., Robinson, T., & Eppich, W. (2017). Coaching the debriefer: Peer coaching to improve debriefing quality in simulation programs. *Simulation in Healthcare: The Journal of the Society for Simulation in Healthcare, 12*(5), 319–325. doi:10.1097/SIH.0000000000000232

Eppich, W., & Cheng, A. (2015). Promoting Excellence and Reflective Learning in Simulation (PEARLS): Development and rationale for a blended approach to health care simulation debriefing. *Simulation in Healthcare: The Journal of the Society for Simulation in Healthcare, 10*(2), 106–115. doi:10.1097/SIH.0000000000000072

Finch, E., Cornwell, P., Nalder, E., & Ward, E. (2015). Uncovering motivators and stumbling blocks: Exploring the clinical research experiences of speech-language pathologists. *International Journal of Speech-Language Pathology, 17*(2), 138–147. doi:10.3109/17549507.2014.930175

Freihoefer, K., Nyberg, G., & Vickery, C. (2013). Clinic exam room design: Present and future. *Health Environments Research & Design Journal, 6*(3), 138–156. doi:10.1177/193758671300600311

Gesler, W., Bell, M., Curtis, S., Hubbard, P., & Francis, S. (2004). Therapy by design: Evaluating the UK hospital building program. *Health Place, 10*(2), 117–128.

Hagan, J., & Walden, M. (2017). Development and evaluation of the barriers to nurse's participation in research questionnaire at a large academic pediatric hospital. *Clinical Nursing Research, 26*(2), 157–175.

Hénard, F., & Roseveare, D. (2012). *Fostering quality teaching in higher education: Policies and practices*. An IMHE Guide for Higher Education Institutions. Retrieved from https://www.scirp.org/(S(i43dyn45teexjx455qlt3d2q))/reference/ReferencesPapers.aspx?ReferenceID=1225873

Holden, R. J., Scanlon, M. C., Patel, N. R., Kaushal, R., Escoto, K. H., Brown, R. L., . . . Karsh, B. T. (2011). A human factors framework and study of the effect of nursing workload on patient safety and employee quality of working life. *BMJ Quality & Safety, 20*(1), 15–24. doi:10.1136/bmjqs.2008.028381

MacPhee, M., Dahinten, S., & Havaei, F. (2017). The impact of heavy perceived nurse workloads on patient nurse outcome. *Administrative Sciences, 7,* 7. doi:10.3390/admsci7010007

Mourshed, M., & Zhao, Y. (2012). Healthcare providers' perception of design factors related to physical environments in hospitals. *Journal of Environmental Psychology, 32*(4), 362–370. doi:10.1016/j.jenvp.2012.06.004

Pittroff, G. E., & Hendricks-Ferguson, V. (2018). Preparing clinical nurses for nursing research. *Journal of Christian Nursing, 35*(1), 38–43. doi:10.1097/CNJ.0000000000000462

Raymond, C., Profetto-McGrath, J., Myrick, F., & Strean, W. B. (2018). Process matters: Successes and challenges of recruiting and retaining participants for nursing education research. *Nurse Education, 43*(2), 92–96. doi:10.1097/NNE.0000000000000423

Scala, E., Price, C., & Day, J. (2016). An integrative review of engaging clinical nurses in nursing research. *Journal of Nursing Scholarship, 48*(4), 423–430. doi:10.1111/jnu.12223

Walsh, K., Ford, K., Morley, C., McLeod, E., McKenzie, D., Chalmers, L., . . . Peterson, G. (2017). The development and implementation of a participatory and solution-focused framework for clinical research: A case example. *Collegian, 24*(4), 331–338. doi:10.1016/j.colegn.2016.06.003

Weller, M. (2014). *The battle for open: How openness won and why it doesn't feel like victory*. London, England: Ubiquity.

White, E. (2012). Challenges that may arise when conducting real-life nursing research. *Nurse Researcher, 19*(4), 15–20. doi:10.7748/nr2012.07.19.4.15.c9219

Woolf, S. H., Zimmerman, E., Haley, A., & Krist, A. H. (2016). In Viewpoint: Authentic engagement of patients and communities can transform research, practice, and policy. *Health Affairs, 35*(4), 590–594.

6 TEAM BUILDING AND INTERPROFESSIONAL COLLABORATION

MARIDEE SHOGREN

INTRODUCTION

DNP students are learning to become skilled healthcare providers and experts in clinical practice but may be especially new to leadership roles. Those enrolled in postbaccalaureate DNP programs may be perceived as novice leaders, especially by project stakeholders who may not yet have an understanding of the DNP degree or its role in clinical practice. Seasoned practitioners attending post-master's DNP programs are more likely to be very comfortable working with patients in a clinical setting; however, they may not have had opportunities to lead projects, present publicly, or tackle systems change. Therefore, most DNP students are emerging leaders.

Numerous texts are available for students to learn about different leadership styles, research which leadership style they most identify with in practice, and even use tools to learn about their own personal leadership qualities. However, in reality, DNP projects move so quickly from brainstorming to dissemination that the student may not have time to fully develop a personal leadership style prior to implementation of the DNP project since most DNP students will often develop their project over three semesters. During that time frame, the DNP student will need to decide who will be on his or her project team, seek advisor approval as well as Institutional Review Board (IRB) approval from the university and the clinical partner if applicable, prepare the timeline for project work and completion, implement the project, evaluate its success, and disseminate the project's findings. The DNP student will not be able to complete these tasks alone and learns very quickly that sharing project responsibilities with his or her team enhances the likelihood of project success.

It will be especially important for the DNP student leader to embrace interprofessional collaboration during the DNP project development and implementation phases. The American Association of Colleges of Nursing (AACN) highlighted interprofessional collaboration in the 2006 *Essentials of Doctoral Education for Advanced Nursing Practice.* In particular, *Essential VI: Interprofessional Collaboration for Improving Patient and Population Health Outcomes* emphasized the fact that DNP members of interprofessional teams should "have advanced preparation in the interprofessional dimension of health care that enable them to facilitate collaborative team functioning and overcome impediments to interprofessional practice." Because effective interprofessional teams function in a highly collaborative fashion and are fluid depending upon the patients' needs, leadership of high performance teams changes. DNP graduates should have preparation in methods of effective team leadership and be prepared to play a central role in establishing interprofessional teams, participating in the work of the team, and assuming leadership of the team when appropriate. "DNP graduates should be able to lead interprofessional teams in the analysis of complex practice and organizational issues" (AACN, 2006, pp. 14–15).

This chapter focuses on the key skills imperative to guide a DNP student through DNP project preparation. Information on developing a positive self-efficacy that can transition to leadership efficacy through implementation of the DNP project is discussed. The concepts of clear communication skills, development of DNP project vision, team building, and team management are presented. Finally, interprofessional competencies and their application to the DNP project team are reviewed. A complementary teacher's guide will assist faculty with introducing some of these important topics to the DNP student.

LEADERSHIP

Leadership is crucial to improving patient outcomes. It establishes the tone for teamwork, provides an environment for team members to ask questions and exchange ideas, and creates a secure sense of belonging for the team (Armstead, Bierman, Bradshaw, Martin, & Wright, 2016). Emerging DNP student leaders should learn to embrace basic leadership skills such as positive self-efficacy, leadership efficacy, and positive communication skills to influence progress toward goal achievement (Whitehead, Dittman, & McNulty, 2017, p 5), in this case, completion of the DNP project.

Initially, DNP students may find it overwhelming to envision themselves as project leaders. It can be equally difficult to engage stakeholders to "buy into" a student project proposal that is new, suggests an evidence-based practice change, or tests an established agency protocol under the guidance of a novice student leader. This may be compounded further by a general lack of understanding the DNP degree and the role of the DNP-prepared nursing leader. It may likewise prove challenging for the DNP student to lead providers and staff from other disciplines if the student is not familiar with their roles and responsibilities. So how does a DNP student begin to tackle this leadership role? One way to conceptualize how the DNP student can develop leadership efficacy may be to apply Bandura's four informational resources: social persuasion, vicarious experiences, mastery, and somatic emotional arousal to identify self-efficacy. Once the DNP student successfully achieves attributes associated with self-efficacy, then they are able to transition and become effective leaders and achieve leadership efficacy (Figure 6.1).

Self-Efficacy

DNP students should be introduced early in their program to the concept of self-efficacy. Self-efficacy is an individual's belief in his or her own abilities to achieve a certain level of performance. Self-efficacy is dynamic and can change with different expectations. DNP students may be more likely to engage in leadership behavior when they believe it will lead to a successful outcome like a successful DNP project. Bandura's Self-Efficacy Theory (as cited in Murphy & Johnson, 2016) identifies four informational sources that can impact a person's self-efficacy (Cziraki, Read, Spence Laschinger, & Wong, 2018).

Mastery experiences, or actually performing a behavior, may be the source most closely linked to the DNP project. However, vicarious experiences (student observation of another person successfully performing a behavior) and social persuasion (telling a person that he or she has the capabilities to master a specific behavior) can also influence the DNP student's achievement of self-efficacy. Finally, somatic and emotional arousal is described as physiologic feedback to people as they make judgments about their self-efficacy. This could be exhibited as pain or anxiety in DNP students; however, this type of information may actually provide DNP students with an opportunity to develop coping skills, which in turn could improve their performance and enhance their leadership growth (Cziraki et al., 2018).

Ideally, the DNP student would use these informational sources to develop a positive self-efficacy and then apply these experiences through leadership of his or her DNP project. Upon completion of the

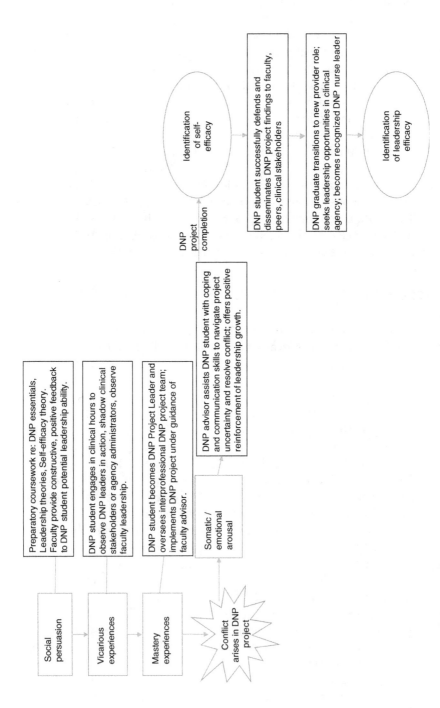

FIGURE 6.1 Application of Bandura's four informational resources to complete a DNP project and achieve leadership efficacy.

DNP project, the DNP student should have the skill set in place to transfer self-efficacy into leadership efficacy (Cziraki et al., 2018).

Leadership Efficacy

Leadership efficacy may actually be one of the most important ingredients in successful leadership and team performance (Murphy & Johnson, 2016). Cziraki et al. (2018) define leadership efficacy as an individual's assessment of his or her knowledge, skills, and abilities needed to lead others effectively. Furthermore, leadership efficacy has been positively associated with leadership performance and "appears to be an important determinant of a person's motivation to lead and desire to pursue a career as a nurse leader" (p. 58). Therefore, the DNP project itself becomes a unique tool to further develop innovative, emerging DNP leaders. Using the knowledge, skills, and abilities achieved through working with other healthcare providers supports the basis for gaining leadership efficacy.

POSITIVE COMMUNICATION SKILLS

Effective communication and teamwork are needed more than ever in the increasingly complex healthcare environment in which DNP leaders practice. Communication plays a critical role in building successful teams, and team communication cannot be overemphasized. Because of the quick turnaround from the conception to evaluation often associated with DNP projects, DNP student leaders need to quickly establish a clear direction for the DNP project and clearly articulate their project vision to the team. Additionally, they must actively listen to team members, expedite conflict resolution, and maintain the course for timely implementation and guide dissemination of project results across many venues (Armstead et al., 2016; Pentland, 2012).

Types of Communication Approaches

Understanding that communication approaches can be influenced by the professional background and respective educational model of clinical training of the DNP leader and each team member, the DNP leader must develop an effective approach that is timely and strategic (Poston, Haney, Kott, & Rutledge, 2017). There are several types of communication skills that may be used during this process; most simply noted are verbal, nonverbal, and written communication skills.

The DNP student must express verbal information in a manner that is not condescending and is clear and concise while avoiding emotional responses like yelling or using an angry tone. Maintaining eye contact with the team while speaking will convey interest and attentiveness. The DNP student should not forget the power of silence as a verbal skill. Nonverbal communication, which actually represents the majority of communication skills, includes appropriate gestures like smiling, relaxed facial expressions, and a posture where the DNP student leans forward slightly and uses open-palm gestures that signal accessibility to the team. Professional dress should be considered as part of the nonverbal domain. Finally, written communication must be accurate and explicit, avoiding the use of jargon and unfamiliar terms that could lead to a lack of understanding among team members (Zaccagnini & White, 2017, pp. 253–256).

Key Elements of Communication

Communication occurs through numerous modalities. Pentland (2012) proposes three key elements of communication: energy, engagement, and exploration. Two of these elements are particularly applicable to DNP project leadership: energy and engagement. Energy is measured by the number and nature of exchanges among team members, with the most valuable form of communication being face-to-face exchange. A strategic communication plan by the DNP student should include some planned face-to-face time on site to communicate with the team implementing the DNP project. Face-to-face time may be best spent on relationship work within the team, staying connected, and resolving conflicts and difficult issues (Craig & McKeown, 2015).

Engagement refers to the distribution of energy among team members. Equal and reasonably high energy among all team members leads to strong engagement and successful outcomes (Pentland, 2012). The DNP student leader will need to balance team engagement with leadership to maintain clear direction and communication of team goals and outcomes (Armstead et al., 2016).

The least valuable form of communication, according to Pentland (2012), includes two forms of written communication, emailing and texting. It can be easy to misinterpret emojis, abbreviated words, and acronyms that are often used in these forms of communication. Tone can also be misunderstood if exclamation points and capitalized letters or phrases are used excessively or inappropriately. However, as long as the language is clear, items like project updates and key positive performance indicators (e.g., recognizing meeting a project milestone) can be shared via these measures or others like group messaging or digital workspaces (Craig & McKeown, 2015).

Two email examples are noted in the following:

- **Poor email example:** ATTENTION DNP PROJECT TEAM! Surveys must be turned in by midnight tonight or we will fall behind schedule on our project timeline. I do not want to see that happen!!! It will jeopardize the entire project.
- **Improved email example:** Hello DNP Project Team! Thank you for your hard work on this DNP project. We have done a great job meeting our timeline goals. Please remember that surveys are due tomorrow night, June 7th, at midnight. If you have not yet completed your survey, you can access the survey at the link included in this email. Please contact me if you have any questions. I appreciate your timely response to this key step in our project work.

TEAM BUILDING

The DNP student leader should be mentally building the project team well before proposing the project concept to key stakeholders. The project team members should include clinical staff or others who are essential to the success of the DNP project. For example, the DNP student should choose a clinical champion employed in the project organization who can assist the student with navigating administration and clinical partners in the workplace. This champion should be someone who understands the organization's IRB and research expectations and be able to assist the student through approval processes. Team members should include clinical staff who can help implement the project, like receptionists, healthcare providers, and information specialists, if this is a clinical quality improvement project, for example. If the DNP student is working on a systematic policy change project, including chief executive officers and administrators may be more applicable. Finally, if the student chooses to conduct a qualitative research project, collaborating with a PhD-prepared nurse to help guide a development of focus group questions and coding would be most appropriate.

Shared Vision

A vision is defined as "forming a detailed mental picture of exactly what you intend to accomplish or produce" (Zaccagnini & White, 2017,

TABLE 6.1 Example of a DNP Project Vision

General Vision Statement	Example of a DNP Project Vision Statement
Improve rates of screening for substance use among females seeking care at a university student health center	This DNP project will implement an alcohol SBI tool into the patient history form used for contraceptive visits in a university student health center

SBI, screening and brief intervention.

Note. The DNP student is encouraged to develop an overall vision and then create a concise statement that clearly depicts the intent of the DNP project.

pp. 405–406). The DNP student leader must be able to imagine the future of the DNP project and inspire others to share in this vision. The DNP student leader should have a clear picture of his or her project and be able to articulate its purpose before bringing it forward to the team for implementation. Without clear identification of the DNP project's shared purpose or vision with the interprofessional team, there may be too many paths to project completion, some of which could be in opposition to the DNP student leader's intent. A shared purpose will provide the needed structure to facilitate project completion (Albert & Priganc, 2014; Zaccagnini & White, 2017, p. 252). As shown in Table 6.1, the DNP project vision statement is concise but provides a clear depiction of the overall goal of the DNP project.

Interprofessional DNP Teams

Healthcare professionals have been called to engage in interprofessional collaboration and practice to solve complex needs within rapidly changing healthcare systems. However, a unique challenge in interprofessional collaboration, such as that encouraged for a DNP project team, is the actual development and function of interprofessional teams for practice and research (Poston et al., 2017). Several team-building concepts are woven throughout the DNP Essentials, including Essential II, which speaks to organizational and systems leadership, and Essential VI, which addresses interprofessional collaboration (AACN, 2006; Armstead et al., 2016).

When designing the DNP project team, it is imperative to select the right personnel and place each in the right position to perform their roles and responsibilities, especially given the short time frame of a DNP project. A proper balance of skills, competencies, practitioner mix, and personalities among team members will afford the DNP student leader the ability to make the most of each team member's background while improving efficiency and effectiveness of the team itself (Armstead et al.,

2016). Team diversity can potentiate creativity and innovation in prob-lem-solving and an ideal team can foster a sense of unity and increase team effectiveness, optimal for achieving a successful DNP project out-come (Beauchamp, McEwan, & Waldhauser, 2017; Poston et al., 2017). A balance of all of these traits may facilitate timely implementation of the DNP project and contribute to a successful project outcome.

A key step of DNP project team building is assembling the most appropriate individuals to move the DNP project forward to comple-tion. Four phases of team formation in small groups were proposed by Tuckman several years ago but are still applicable and a good fit for for-mation of a DNP project team. These phases include forming, storming, norming, and performing (Craig & McKeown, 2015; Poston et al., 2017; Tuckman, 1965; Zaccagnini & White, 2017), and by understanding these components, the DNP student can be more successful in team building.

Forming

DNP students, as responsible leaders, must focus on building effective relationships with a network of stakeholders. They need to encourage the entire team to collaborate and work toward a shared vision and do so over a relatively short period of time (Albert & Priganc, 2014). During the forming phase, the DNP student must identify who will have a vested interest in the project and should include individuals who can partner with the academic institution. This will facilitate any institutional bar-riers and assist the student in navigating the nuances of the project set-ting along with those who will be implementing the actual project. The DNP leader should use this phase for orientation and to clarify the roles for each member involved in the project (Tuckman, 1965; Zaccagnini & White, 2017, p. 454). Early on, it will be important to identify the stake-holders who will be key players in sustaining the project work after its completion and when the DNP student is no longer directly involved.

It may be quite helpful to introduce assessment and project man-agement tools during this phase. A personal assessment tool, like the discprofile (2019, https://www.discprofile.com), used to improve work productivity, teamwork, and communication, or the Myers–Briggs Type Indicator® (https://www.myersbriggs.org/my-mbti-personality-type/mbti-basics/) personality inventory, used to better understand person-ality preferences, may act as icebreaker tools and provide foundational insight into how the group will work together or where strengths/weaknesses may lie. They may also accelerate transition through the storming phase and lead to a more productive performing stage for interprofessional teams (Poston et al., 2017). Additional icebreaker ideas to start team building can be found on websites like MindTools® (www.mindtools.com/pages/article/newLDR_76.htm).

Tools like a Gantt chart (www.gantt.com) or workflow diagram can provide structure for the team by clearly laying out deadlines, documenting milestones, and clarifying expectations. These tools may also help the team stay focused as internal and external factors constantly change and can impact the work of the project (Albert & Priganc, 2014). The DNP leader can use these tools to demonstrate directive leadership skills and instill confidence in the project team.

Storming

This second phase is characterized by conflict and division around interpersonal concerns with concurrent emotional responses (Tuckman, 1965). The DNP leader may feel intimated or challenged during this phase, and it will be important to have resources available to navigate any conflicts. Conflicts are inevitable as team members compete for authority, try to defend personal positions, and challenge the DNP project plan and potentially the DNP student leader. However, conflict is also vital for interprofessional team effectiveness and can lead to positive group functioning depending on leadership style (Zaccagnini & White, 2017, p. 258). Rather than avoiding conflict, the DNP leader can learn to use collaborative conflict management tools to find solutions.

One practical conflict management tool is known as the "Walk in the Woods" guide. The Walk in the Woods is a four-step process to structure interest-based negotiation among stakeholders and is designed to build confidence. Because people only truly embrace solutions that they help create, the DNP student leader should include all DNP project members in this quick intervention to manage conflict. Steps include:

- Self-interests: Articulate your self-interests and actively hear those of others; distinguish legitimate "self" from "selfish" interest
- Enlarged interests: Identify points of agreement and points of disagreement among stakeholders to gather a multidimensional view of the problem and reframe
- Enlightened interests: Explore and/or invent options and assess which options generate agreement. Prioritize and focus on solutions that could generate agreement
- Aligned interests: Seek mutually beneficial solutions and generate buy-in. Resolve. Agree. Commit. Move forward (Dorn, Marcus, & McNulty, 2013; Marcus, Dorn, Henderson, & Ashkenazi, 2008).

DNP student leaders can also draw on the concepts of emotional intelligence to enhance their leadership skills. Recognizing their own emotions, maintaining composure during challenging situations, offering adaptability and flexibility to facilitate change, and remaining sensitive and empathetic to the team will be a direct reflection of their leadership skills and help build positive relationships on the team (Zaccagnini & White, 2017, p. 258).

Norming

This phase generates the team's commitment to the project tasks and goals. Team cohesiveness develops here as new standards evolve and new roles are adopted (Tuckman, 1965). As the team settles into implementation of the project, the DNP leader will continuously need to encourage collaboration and mutual problem-solving (Zaccagnini & White, 2017, p. 459). Continued utilization of conflict management tools like "Walk in the Woods" (Marcus et al., 2008) during this phase of collaboration provides the student with a tangible method for ongoing problem resolution.

Performing

This is the final phase of team formation. Structural issues have been resolved, and member roles become flexible, functional, and supportive as the team works to complete project tasks and goals (Tuckman, 1965). As the team works toward project completion, the DNP leader will need to remember that team members often hold responsibilities outside of the work of the DNP project. It is important that the DNP student leader keeps the project on task, refers back to the workflow chart, and delegates as necessary but remains responsible for the project's overall completion (Zaccagnini & White, 2017, p. 459). Celebrating project milestones should not be forgotten and the DNP student should provide positive feedback to the team for their participation. This is an ideal time to utilize a form of written communication, like a text or email, to thank the project team for the hard work that has been accomplished to date and remind them that project completion is near.

Team Management

Equally as important to completing the DNP project through a shared vision with the ideal interprofessional team is the concept of successful team management. Successful management of the DNP project can only occur through work that is planned, organized, and consistent. The importance of clear communication and two team management tools, a Gantt chart or workflow diagram to manage deadlines and document milestones and a conflict resolution tool like "Walk in the Woods" to problem-solve, have already been introduced in this chapter. Other team management strategies that may be valuable to the DNP student leader include appropriate delegation of tasks, setting ground rules for meetings, adherence to an agenda, clear and early notification of location and time of meetings, and a record of meeting minutes made readily available to team members.

The DNP student may also need to manage non-healthcare professionals like receptionists, informaticians, and billing and coding staff. Appropriately applied communication skills as previously discussed will also be valuable with these groups. The DNP student leader should include these professionals in training sessions and communication regarding project updates and changes. Inclusion in these areas has been reported to lead to persisting changes in knowledge and behavior (Albardiaz, 2012), which ideally could enhance DNP project sustainability within the organization.

INTERPROFESSIONAL COLLABORATION

Finally, the DNP student leader must remember that interprofessional teams tend to have complex structures. The DNP student will have a nursing background; however, other members of the team may come from varied disciplines, including those with a nonmedical background (Armstead et al., 2016). Many DNP students will have been introduced to interprofessional concepts through previous nursing coursework; however, faculty should reaffirm these ideas with the DNP student leader and encourage interprofessional collaboration during the DNP project.

The Interprofessional Education Collaborative (IPEC) was formed in 2009 when six national associations of schools of health professions made a collaborative effort to advance interprofessional learning experiences for health professional students. Their goal then, and now, was to prepare future health professionals for team-based patient care and ultimately improve population health outcomes. Their recommendations were first published in 2011. In 2016, IPEC updated its core competencies to better reflect a stand-alone domain of interprofessional collaboration and increase focus on the Institute for Healthcare Improvement (IHI) "Triple Aim" approach to healthcare (IPEC, 2016). The "Triple Aim" approach refers to the simultaneous pursuit of improving the patient experience of care, improving the health of populations, and reducing the per capita cost of healthcare. DNP projects are perfect opportunities to improve patient outcomes by utilizing the "Triple Aim" approach. Application of the updated four IPEC core competencies, as well as select subcompetencies, is integral to implementation of the DNP project and is summarized in Table 6.2.

TABLE 6.2 IPEC Core Competencies and Application to a DNP Project

IPEC Core Competency	IPEC Subcompetency	Application to DNP Project
Values/Ethics for Interprofessional Practice: Work with individuals of other professions to maintain a climate of mutual respect and shared values	V/E6: Develop a trusting relationship with other team members	DNP leader gets to know team members through icebreaker activities and use of personal assessment tools to evaluate individual skills/personalities
Roles/Responsibilities: Use the knowledge of one's own role and those of other professions to appropriately assess and address the healthcare needs of patients and to promote and advance the health of populations	R/R6: Communicate with team members to clarify each member's responsibility in executing components of a public health intervention	DNP leader introduces a workflow diagram to clearly identify project milestones and a responsible team member for each task
Interprofessional Communication: Communicate with patients, families, communities, and professionals in health and other fields in a responsive and responsible manner that supports a team approach to the promotion and maintenance of health and the prevention and treatment of disease	CC1: Choose effective communication tools and techniques, including information systems and communication technologies, to facilitate discussions and interactions that enhance team function	DNP leader uses a combination of oral and written communication strategies like face-to-face meetings with agendas and record of minutes and emails to provide project updates
Teams and Teamwork: Apply relationship-building values and the principles of team dynamics to perform effectively in different team roles to plan, deliver, and evaluate patient/population-centered care and population health programs and policies that are safe, timely, efficient, effective, and equitable	TT5: Apply leadership practices that support collaborative practice and team effectiveness	DNP leader delegates responsibilities as needed, remains cognizant of team members' time constraints and responsibilities outside of DNP project, adheres to workflow diagram, and celebrates milestones with team

IPEC, Interprofessional Education Collaborative.

Source: Adapted from Interprofessional Education Collaborative. (2016). *Core competencies for interprofessional collaborative practice: 2016 update*. Washington, DC: Author.

The DNP student's ability to engage with all members of the DNP project team is enhanced through application of the IPEC core competencies. While these competencies provide a framework for effective collaboration within a structured project, they also guide the DNP student though an exercise in active learning that demonstrates how true collaborative practice translates innovative strategies into improved patient outcomes and healthcare system change.

SUMMARY

In summary, there are several key concepts and skills that will benefit an emerging DNP leader. Even though the time frame for implementing a DNP project is relatively short, applying the appropriate concepts at each stage of project preparation will reinforce the DNP student's understanding of leadership. Faculty members have a responsibility to provide DNP students with opportunities to foster the development of self-efficacy and provide positive reinforcement to DNP students as their leadership skills evolve. Including concepts of clear communication skills, shared visions, and team building will translate into well-managed and successful DNP projects. Finally, instilling DNP students with the knowledge of interprofessional teams and the importance of interprofessional collaboration provides a foundation for continued collaborative practice in a variety of healthcare settings. Interprofessional practice is truly the core work that will improve patient outcomes.

APPLICATION EXERCISES: TEAM BUILDING, LEADERSHIP, AND INTERPROFESSIONAL COLLABORATION

Introduction

The IPEC (2019) was founded in 2009 to address the need to form a consistent, collaborative health profession organization that would provide future health professionals with the core competencies to provide team-based care of patients and improve population health outcomes. The collaborative consisted of representatives from nursing, dentistry, medicine, pharmacy, and public health. As a result, in 2011, the "Core Competencies for Interprofessional Collaborative Practice" was developed as a guide to educate future health professionals (IPEC, 2019).

The interprofessional collaboration domain as recognized by educators has been used for curriculum design and mapping of content indigenous to the interprofessional model. The four competency areas of interprofessional practice that were developed included: values/ethics, roles/responsibilities, interprofessional communication, and teams and teamwork. An important aspect of each of these overall domains included the subcompetencies specific to safe patient care. Within each of the core competencies and subcompetencies feature the following desired principles: patient- and family-centered (hereafter termed "patient-centered"); community and population oriented; relationship focused; process oriented; linked to learning activities, educational strategies, and behavioral assessments that are developmentally appropriate for the learner; able to be integrated across the learning continuum; sensitive to the systems context and applicable across practice settings; applicable across professions; stated in language common and meaningful across the professions; and outcome driven IPEC, 2019).

The following overall four core competencies continue to be used as a guideline for providing safe interprofessional clinical practice.

- *Competency 1:* Work with individuals of other professions to maintain a climate of mutual respect and shared values (Values/Ethics for Interprofessional Practice).
- *Competency 2:* Use the knowledge of one's own role and those of other professions to appropriately assess and address the healthcare needs of patients and to promote and advance the health of populations (Roles/Responsibilities).
- *Competency 3:* Communicate with patients, families, communities, and professionals in health and other fields in a responsive and responsible manner that supports a team approach to the promotion and maintenance of health and the prevention and treatment of disease (Interprofessional Communication).
- *Competency 4:* Apply relationship-building values and the principles of team dynamics to perform effectively in different team roles to plan, deliver, and evaluate patient/population-centered care and population health programs and policies that are safe, timely, efficient, effective, and equitable (Teams and Teamwork); see IPEC (2019).
- The subcategories for each of the core competencies are listed in tables available online (nebula.wsimg. com/2f68a39520b03336b41038c370497473?AccessKeyId= DC06780E69ED19E2B3A5&disposition=0&alloworigin=1).

Case Presentation

Roberto Garzon, a 27-year-old Hispanic immigrant, comes to the free clinic in rural Georgia after being refused a day job because he "coughed" too much. The desk clerk noted that Mr. Garzon could not speak English, so she called a volunteer (Maria) over who was bilingual. Mr. Garzon stated to Maria that he was told to come to the clinic to get rid of his cough and to be sure that he was fit to work. The nurse tech (Anna) obtained Mr. Garzon's vital signs while Maria was present so that he would feel welcomed and not be frightened. While Anna was obtaining his vital signs, Mr. Garzon had several episodes of productive coughing. His vital signs were: blood pressure: 140/88; pulse: 102; resp: 24 and temp: 99.0. Anna obtained the following information from Mr. Garzon: he had been working as a day laborer for the past 2 weeks and had been exposed to several other day laborers who also were coughing. He smokes 1 pk/day cigarettes and is able to eat at the homeless shelter in a nearby church.

Medical History

NP Hazel walks in and asks Maria to stay with her while she completes a history and physical exam. Hazel asks the following questions:

- How has your appetite been?
- Have you been more tired than usual?
- Have you had any chest pains?
- How long have you been coughing?
- Do you wake up at night with the cough?
- Have you had any night sweats?
- Do you cough anything up?
- What do you take to relieve the cough?
- Have you ever had any immunizations?

Hazel noted the following: Mr. Garzon has had the cough for over 8 weeks that has gotten progressively worse and that he has been coughing up sputum that has become more frequent. He has not been able to sleep through the night since he wakes up coughing or hears others coughing at the homeless shelter. He has no access to over-the-counter medications nor has he been seen by any other healthcare provider. Hazel suspects that Mr. Garzon has not been immunized and is suspicious about his constant cough.

Physical Exam

Physical exam revealed the following:

- Malnourished, diaphoretic, and pale 27-year-old male
- HEENT: throat slightly reddened and irritated
- Lymph system: positive submaxillary lymphadenopathy
- Neuro exam: unremarkable
- Lungs: rhonchi both lower lobes, with expiratory wheezing
- Abdomen: unremarkable
- Extremities: unremarkable

Medical and Laboratory Tests
- Complete blood count (CBC)
- Urine
- Sputum
- Chest x-ray
- Tuberculosis (TB) tine test

Laboratory and Chest X-Ray Results
- CBC, elevated white blood cell (WBC) count, Hct, Hb, normal
- Urine: negative
- Sputum: pending
- Chest X-ray: tubercular nodules sporadically noted 1 to 2 cm each lung

Diagnosis
R/O active TB

Discussion With Patient
With Maria present, Hazel met with Mr. Garzon to review his diagnosis and discuss a plan of care. Hazel explained that he had TB and that it was a serious infectious disease and that it was important that he stick to a treatment plan so that he could get better. Hazel stated that he would need to be isolated from other people so that he would not infect others. She stated that a social worker (Evelyn) would assist him to obtain a place to live outside of the homeless shelter. Hazel explained that he would need to take the medications that would be given to him today and that it would be important that he come back to the clinic for follow-up medical care. Additionally, Hazel explained that the nurse from the health department would be contacting him to check on him to ensure he is taking his medication and getting his health needs met. Hazel provided the medical treatment plan and follow-up services to Mr. Garzon.

Medications
- Isoniazid (INH)
- Rifampin (RIF)

- Ethambutol (EMB)
- Pyrazinamide (PZA)
- Specific information about the dosing regimen can be found at: www.cdc.gov/tb/topic/treatment/tbdisease.htm

Follow-Up
- Report patient occurrence to local health department (name of patient and contact information)
- Provide immediate treatment medications
- Arrange 2-week follow-up for a clinic appointment
- Notify the local homeless shelter to bring other clients in for testing for TB
- Notify the clinic social worker to obtain alternate housing to isolate patient
- Referral to infectious disease doctor

Application Exercise Questions

Part I: Application of IPEC core competencies and subcategories. Based on the case presentation, fill in the following chart listing the IPEC subcategories and exemplars from the clinical case presentation that support the overall IPEC competencies and subcategories. Answers for the table can be found in Chapter 11, Application Exercise Answer Keys.

IPEC Core Competency	IPEC Subcategories	Case Study Exemplars
Competency 1: Values/Ethics for Interprofessional Practice		
Competency 2: Roles/ Responsibilities		
Competency 3: Interprofessional Communication		
Competency 4: Teams and Teamwork		

Part II: Based on the aforementioned case study, address the following questions. Suggested answers can be found in Chapter 11, Application Exercise Answer Keys.

1. How would you plan the healthcare needs for a transient patient population when using the IPEC categories and subcategories?
2. What steps would you take to address the cultural needs of a patient population?
3. Discuss the systemic changes needed to provide effective quality patient care.

REFERENCES

Albardiaz, R. (2012). Communication skills and team-building for receptionists and ancillary staff. *Education for Primary Care, 23*(1), 44–46.

Albert, D., & Priganc, D. (2014). Building a team through a strategic planning process. *Nursing Administration Quarterly, 38*(3), 238–247. doi:10.1097/NAQ.0000000000000036

American Association of Colleges of Nursing. (2006). *The essentials of doctoral education for advanced nursing practice.* Retrieved from http://www.aacnnursing.org/DNP/DNP-Essentials

Armstead, C., Bierman, D., Bradshaw, P., Martin, T., & Wright, K. (2016). Groups vs teams: Which one are you leading? *Nurse Leader, 14*(3), 179–182. doi:10.1016/j.mnl.2016.03.006

Beauchamp, M., McEwan, D., & Waldhauser, K. (2017). Team building: Conceptual, methodological, and applied considerations. *Current Opinion in Psychology, 16*, 114–117. doi:10.1016/j.copsyc.2017.02.031

Craig, M., & McKeown, D. (2015). How to build effective teams in healthcare. *Nursing Times, 111*(14), 16–18.

Cziraki, K., Read, E., Spence Laschinger, H., & Wong, C. (2018). Nurses' leadership self-efficacy, motivation, and career aspirations. *Leadership in Health Services, 31*(1), 47–61. doi:10.1108/LHS-02-2017-0003

discprofile. (2019). Retrieved from https://www.discprofile.com

Dorn, B., Marcus, L., & McNulty, E. (2013, October). Four steps to resolving conflicts in health care. *Harvard Business Review.* Retrieved from https://hbr.org/2013/10/four-steps-to-resolving-conflicts-in-health-care

Gantt chart software. (2019). *What is a Gantt chart?* Retrieved from https://www.gantt.com

Interprofessional Education Collaborative. (2019). *Core competencies for interprofessional collaborative practice: 2016 update.* Retrieved from: https://nebula.wsimg.com/2f68a39520b03336b41038c370497473?AccessKeyId=DC06780E69ED19E2B3A5&disposition=0&alloworigin=1

Marcus, L., Dorn, B., Henderson, J., & Ashkenazi, I. (2008). *Linking multidimensional problems to complex, multi-party solutions. The Walk in the Woods: A guide for meta-leaders.* Retrieved from www.hcna.net/pdf/Workbook_WalkintheWoods.pdf

MindTools Ltd. (2019). *Ice breakers: Easing group contribution.* Retrieved from www.mindtools.com/pages/article/newLDR_76.htm

Murphy, S., & Johnson, K. (2016). Leadership and leader developmental self-efficacy: Their role in enhancing leader development efforts. *New Directions for Student Leadership, 2016*(149), 73–84. doi:10.1002/yd.20163

The Myers & Briggs Foundation. (2019). MBTI® basics. Retrieved from https://www.myersbriggs.org/my-mbti-personality-type/mbti-basics/

Pentland, A. (2012). The new science of building great teams: The chemistry of high-performing groups is no longer a mystery. *Harvard Business Review,* pp. 61–70.

Poston, R., Haney, T., Kott, K., & Rutledge, C. (2017). Interprofessional team performance optimized: Enhance development with behavioral profiles. *Nursing Management, 48,* 37–43 doi:10.1097/01.NUMA.0000520722.55679.7c

Tuckman, B. (1965). Developmental sequence in small groups. *Psychological Bulletin, 63*(6), 384–399. doi:10.1037/h0022100

Whitehead, D., Dittman P., & McNulty, D. (2017). *Leadership and the advanced practice nurse: The future of a changing health-care environment.* Philadelphia, PA: F.A. Davis Company.

Zaccagnini, M., & White, K. (2017). *The doctor of nursing practice essentials: A new model for advanced practice nursing* (3rd ed.). Burlington, MA: Jones & Bartlett Learning.

7   DEBRIEFING THE CLINICAL STAFF

MARY WYCKOFF

INTRODUCTION

Achieving a DNP degree will provide education and preparation to facilitate your ability to implement high levels of change with demanding expectations for a scholarly approach in achieving these goals. Practice-focused programs place emphasis on practice gaps and understanding how to fix the problems. Actually making the change is the difficulty in the implementation of a clinical project. As the leader in these situations, facilitating the understanding of the DNP project, while implementing the process, is critical. Integrating the DNP project into the daily activities of clinical practice provides simplification of ensuring the change is implemented and sustainable. Ensuring sustainability can be instituted by critical debriefing sessions that provide a feedback mechanism for all learners. It is important to conduct debriefing sessions with clinical staff, from each of the clinical settings that contribute to the project, especially since they interact with patients and can have important recommendations that may not be expected by the student. This chapter focuses on the following steps: (a) understanding debriefing and the DNP project; (b) clinical practice learning styles and debriefing; (c) application of Miller's pyramid for assessment; and (d) facilitator principles for debriefing sessions. Finally, this chapter provides examples as to how to apply the theoretical concepts of learning to the application of a debriefing session in a clinical practice setting.

UNDERSTANDING DEBRIEFING AND THE DNP PROJECT

The goal of the DNP project is to facilitate clinical care concepts that are based on scientific data that increase quality and safety of patient care while integrating practice from multiple disciplines. DNP students will be successful in conducting their clinical project by understanding the TeamSTEPPS (Quality and Safety Education for Nurses [QSEN], 2018) model when working with clinical teams. The key principles of the TeamSTEPPS (AHRQ, 2019) model include the team's infrastructure, communication among team members, leadership, situation monitoring, and mutual support of each team member. The development of the DNP project must incorporate the team concepts to facilitate the "buy-in" from the clinical individuals who will implement the components of the project. Furthermore, the task force on the implementation of the DNP (American Association of Colleges of Nursing [AACN], 2015a) recommended that the content for DNP projects should include the following areas:

- Focus on a change that impacts healthcare outcomes
- Have a system (micro-, meso-, or macrolevel) or population/ aggregate focus
- Demonstrate implementation in the appropriate arena or area of practice
- Include a plan for sustainability (e.g., financial, systems or political realities, not only theoretical abstractions)
- Include an evaluation of processes and/or outcomes (formative or summative)
- Provide a foundation for future practice scholarship

Group/team projects can be a valuable experience to help prepare DNP graduates to function in interprofessional and intraprofessional teams since today this is an expectation in clinical practice as well as in the future models of healthcare delivery. These situations often present challenges, particularly for student evolution and development. When working on projects that are in the student's area of practice and the project goals are consistent with the program, students should anticipate that an inter/intracollaborative clinical enviroment will facilitate in the development of their project.

Guidelines for the entire project as well as for individual evaluation and overall contributions to the project should be developed and shared with the students prior to the initiation of the project. Each member of the group must meet all expectations of planning, implementation, and evaluation of the project, and be evaluated accordingly. Each student must have a leadership role in at least one component of the project and be held accountable for a deliverable (AACN, 2015b). The following serve as illustrative examples:

- The student serves as a vital member of an interprofessional team, implementing and evaluating a component of a larger project.
- Students work on the same project; for example, improving handwashing, across multiple units within the same organization or across multiple organizations.
- Students focus on different aspects of improving diabetic outcomes of care by meeting criteria for guidelines for diabetes care such as eye exams, time frames for HbA1C screening, and foot care.
- Students analyze and implement changes in state immunization policies to improve access to immunizations and increase immunization rates.

These topics clearly define practice gaps and would be implemented as inter-/intradisciplinary team projects requiring full evaluation and debriefing for successful implementation, sustainability, and evolution for ongoing collaboration.

The DNP student projects will facilitate change in the healthcare environment only when the plan for sustainability is sound and incorporates a debriefing capability. Debriefing has been clearly researched in war, airline/crew debriefing situations, posttraumatic situations, codes, and simulation. Understanding debriefing is critical to implement and sustain the project outcomes and allows for the natural evolution of project development. According to Fillion, Clements, Averill, and Virgil (2002), the beginning of debriefing sessions was seen in the military during World War II. The army's chief historian Brigadier General Marshall performed the first Historical Group Debriefing where the soldiers discussed the events of combat, their emotions, and decisions. The outcome was termed "Spiritual Purging," facilitating psychological benefits when discussing the outcomes of different battles as to how to survive and improve.

There are structured and supported debriefing models. The National Aeronautics and Space Administration (NASA), for example, utilizes crew resource by performing a summary and evaluation of the operations. The American Heart Association gathers, analyzes, and summarizes data from surviving victims of heart attacks and strokes. Furthermore a three-dimensional model related to debriefing diffuses the idea, discovers the information, deepens understanding, and summarizes the impact. By using these models of debriefing, teams can further develop ways to make improvements associated with problems or issues that occurred during a mission.

Integration of debriefing sessions as a result of the DNP project into the mainstream of the daily routine is critical to success. This approach seems logical since it provides avenues to change clinical practice. An interdisciplinary debriefing discussion about changing the rate of hospital infection rates was most successful when implemented into the electronic medical record (EMR). As an example, the national move to zero hospital infection rates and the daily evaluation of central line access was most successful when it became a daily check in the EMR with a trigger to the healthcare providers to ensure this was assessed daily (QSEN, 2018). Thus, it makes sense to incorporate debriefing sessions into DNP projects, especially since they encourage change processes in the clinical area.

LEARNING STYLES AND DEBRIEFING

Understanding how clinical staff learn during debriefing sessions can best be described by David Kolb's theory of learning. David Kolb (1984) established learning styles incorporating the experiential learning theory, which works on two separate levels incorporating a four-stage cycle of learning and four separate learning styles that integrate the learner's internal cognitive processes. These abstract concepts have a flexibility that focuses on the development of learning new concepts through new experiences. The new experiences are enhanced by the debriefing process. Kolb noted that "learning is the process whereby knowledge is created through the transformation of experience" (Kolb, 1984, p. 38). An understanding of how learning occurs as a result of the experience is the foundation of Kolb's theory and provides the basis of the debriefing process.

Experiential learning style theory is typically represented by a four-stage learning cycle in which the learner "touches all the bases" (Figure 7.1).

Application of Kolb's experiential learning theory to the DNP project may include an understanding of each of the four-stage learning cycles when reviewing a clinical situation. Exemplars for each component of Kolb's learning theory as applied to the clinical environment may include:

- **Concrete experiences** (a new clinical experience or a situation in clinical practice is encountered, or a reinterpretation of existing clinical experience)

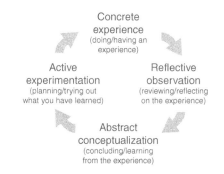

FIGURE 7.1 Kolb's experiential learning theory.

Source: From McLeod, S. (2017). Kolb's learning styles and experiential learning cycle. Retrieved from https://www.simplypsychology.org/learning-kolb.html

- **Reflective observation of the new experience** (of particular importance are any inconsistencies between experience and understanding of the clinical situation)
- **Abstract conceptualization** (reflection gives rise to a new clinical idea or a modification of an existing abstract clinical concept). This component facilitates the debriefing portion of the cycle
- **Active experimentation** (the learner applies ideas to the clinical environment and tries out the results; Kolb and Kolb, 2005)

Effective learning styles occur when a person progresses through a cycle of four stages: (a) having a concrete experience; (b) observation of and reflection on that experience; (c) formation of an abstract concept (analysis) and generalizations (conclusions); (d) the concept and generalizations are then (through debriefing) used to test hypotheses in future situations or new experiences (Figure 7.2).

The application of an effective learning style related to the DNP project may include an interdisciplinary clinical simulation related to medical errors as a result of miscommunication and negative patient outcomes. For example, the identification of the wrong patient, wrong medication, and cardiac or respiratory arrest resulting from the medication error and debriefing discussions related to the experience assist the learner in the understanding of the impact of the clinical error. Reflection about the experience to all team members, conceptualization of how to change the scenario, and testing how change could be implemented would be discussed among all clinical staff during a debriefing session. The facilitator of the debriefing discussion would

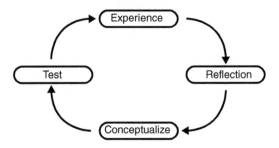

FIGURE 7.2 Effective learning: a four-stage cycle.

Source: From McLeod, S. (2017). Kolb's learning styles and experiential learning cycle. Retrieved from https://www.simplypsychology.org/learning-kolb.html

assist in the discussions of the clinical issue and provide examples of accommodation, diverging, assimilation, and converging. Thus, the effective learning style only occurs when a learner can execute all four stages of the model.

Kolb's learning theory (1984) sets out four distinct learning styles, which further expands the understanding of how learners think. The four learning styles are based on a four-stage learning cycle. During a debriefing session, an integrated approach to learning occurs as a result of the clinical experience. An understanding of Kolb's learning theory as it applies to the debriefing process may include the application of Kolb's two continuums. For example, a typical presentation of Kolb's two continuums is that the east–west axis is called the **processing continuum** (how we approach a task) and the north–south axis is called the **perception continuum** (our emotional response or how we think or feel about it), which has been compared to debriefing sessions (Kolb & Kolb, 2005). It is the integration of each of the processing and perception continuums that can facilitate a successful debriefing session. Kolb (1984) suggests that for effective learning to occur, the learner should execute all four stages of the model (Figure 7.3).

Kolb believed that we cannot perform both variables on a single axis at the same time (e.g., think and feel). Our learning style is a product of these two choice decisions, which is facilitated through the debriefing process as we actualize and correlate this process (Kolb & Kolb, 2005).

The application of Kolb's learning styles to the debriefing process includes the decision-making process about a clinical situation and the discussion about the clinical situation. The discussion may include the underlying factors that occurred during the clinical encounter. Examples may include time, clinical staff involved, communication, medication

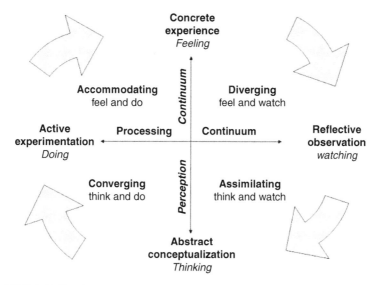

FIGURE 7.3 Kolb's four-stage model of learning.

Source: From McLeod, S. (2017). Kolb's learning styles and experiential learning cycle. Retrieved from https://www.simplypsychology.org/learning-kolb.html

given, status of patient, or interdepartment issues. The debriefing process assists in the overall analysis of the clinical situation, and understanding how we learn and make choices will help health professionals internalize the clinical situation and avoid future negative outcomes.

A further understanding of the construction of Kolb's learning styles can be demonstrated by using a 2 x 2 matrix that highlights the four learning styles and the terminology associated with the four learning styles (Table 7.1).

TABLE 7.1 Matrix of Kolb's Terminology and Four Learning Styles

	Active Experimentation (Doing)	Reflective Observation (Watching)
Concrete Experience (Feeling)	Accommodating (CE/AE)	Diverging (CE/RO)
Abstract Conceptualization (Thinking)	Converging (AC/AE) (Debriefing)	Assimilating (AC/RO) (Implementation of the outcomes of the debrief)

Source: From McLeod, S. (2017). Kolb's learning styles and experiential learning cycle. Retrieved from https://www.simplypsychology.org/learning-kolb.html

Kolb and Kolb's (2005) terminology for the four learning styles includes diverging, assimilating, converging (debriefing), and accommodating (implementing the outcomes of the debriefing). Descriptions of the four learning styles are important in the understanding of this learning style, and how it pertains to the debriefing model in clinical practice has been listed in the following.

Diverging (feeling and watching—CE/RO)

- Diverging involves seeing from different perspectives and viewing concrete situations from several different viewpoints. This may be considered the brainstorming portion of the project.

Assimilating (watching and thinking—AC/RO)

- Assimilating involves a concise, logical approach. Ideas and concepts are developed into a practical protocol for implementation and practice. The focus is on effectiveness and a logical approach.

Converging (doing and thinking—AC/AE)

- Converging involves the solving of problems, and learning is used to find solutions to practical issues. This is the actual debriefing phase in which new ideas are used to simulate and to work with practical applications.

Accommodating (doing and feeling—CE/AE)

- Accommodating learning style is implementing and carrying out the solutions found in the debriefing phase through feelings and logical analysis.

The importance of Kolb's model as it relates to the understanding of clinical debriefing scenarios is important for the facilitators of a debriefing session. For example, it is important for the facilitator to take the time for the learners to process their thinking as they reflect on the experience. During reflection (divergence), learners may be processing their feelings about the experience and thinking about the possible outcomes associated with the experience. Additionally, during the reflective process, the clinical staff may be assimilating their thoughts, which includes conceptualizing the processes that may have occurred. Furthermore, the facilitator of the debriefing session would be cognizant of understanding that the clinical staff would need time to conceptualize and actively experiment with other options associated with the incident. Discussions may include how clinicians think, feel, and do (convergence, accommodating) their clinical tasks and reflect about what could have been done differently. An understanding of Kolb's integration model of learning and learning styles provides the structure needed for the facilitators of debriefing sessions and affords the skills necessary for a successful clinical debriefing session.

MILLER'S PYRAMID FOR ASSESSMENT

From the outset, the DNP student should consider how to be actively involved in the clinical project and any debriefing issues that may occur. For example, it is important that the DNP student understand the major key stakeholders, staff, and other clinical providers who will be involved in the implementation of the DNP project in the clinical facility. Using Miller's pyramid for assessment (Miller, 1990), which focuses on the concepts of knows, knows how, shows, and does, provides a framework for incorporating best practices within the change process in a clinical setting. More importantly, clinicians as learners will incorporate the change process best by actively participating in brief lectures, group discussions, and small group practices during debriefing sessions.

Though the focus of the pyramid is on clinical-based scenarios, this may be implemented to evaluate the stages of competency and ability for the clinical staff or graduate students participating with the project to accept change. An example of how to use Miller's Competence Pyramid has been provided in the following.

Exemplar: *DNP problem, intervention, comparison, outcome, and time (PICOT)*
Will the implementation of Situation, Background, Assessment, and Recommendation (SBAR) communication with the nursing staff at General Hospital on 5 East increase the communication of information, compared to the current standard of practice as demonstrated by a decrease in incident reports due to miscommunication over 12 weeks?

Problem: Miscommunication as demonstrated by increase in incident reports
Intervention: Implementation of SBAR communication process
Comparison: Current standard of practice
Outcome: Use of SBAR communication and decrease in incident reports regarding miscommunication
Time frame: 12 weeks
Debriefing: Implementation of a debriefing process to ensure the stakeholders comprehend the project outcomes and the rationale for change based on the use of Miller's Competence Pyramid for evaluation of knowledge comprehension and critical thinking to facilitate sustainability of change

The application of Miller's Competence Pyramid, descriptions, and examples of evaluation are listed in the following.

KNOWS forms the base of the pyramid and the foundation for building competence for the project change.

- Ex1: Learner is assessed his or her knowledge of the SBAR process by demonstrating the change process through implementation of the SBAR communication process.
- Ex2: Learner knows how to implement and demonstrate the process.
- Ex3: Learner knows the indications, contraindications, and risks associated with miscommunication.

KNOWS HOW uses knowledge in the acquisition, analysis, and interpretation of data and the development of a plan.

- Ex1: Learner evaluates his or her own SBAR process and evaluates the clarity of communication.
- Ex2: Learner knows how to provide the critical information regarding a patient encounter, utilize history, physical exam, and diagnostic test data to facilitate clear communication.
- Ex3: Learner knows, given a simulated appropriate clinical scenario, to provide the project change SBAR communication.

SHOWS HOW requires the learner to demonstrate the integration of knowledge and skills into successful clinical performance.

- Ex1: Learner demonstrates how he or she would respond to a standardized patient's communication process.
- Ex2: Learner shows how to develop and implement a patient SBAR communication process.
- Ex3: Learner shows how to complete an SBAR communication process.

DOES focuses on the project change and consistent implementation of the desired change process supported through the debriefing process.

- Ex1: Learner is assessed through case scenarios and debriefing.
- Ex2: Learner demonstrates the ability to evaluate the communication process and the outcomes of the change.
- Ex3: Learner comprehends and understands the statistical change process. (Miller, 1990)

By using Miller's Competence Pyramid through various debriefing clinical scenarios, the clinical staff could be guided by the DNP facilitator to explore a variety of educational learning styles that assist in the change process. Adaptation of new educational models that have been used during the debriefing sessions assists staff to transition through potential clinical events and provides new skills that can be used to identify potential problems during routine clinical practice.

FACILITATOR PRINCIPLES FOR DEBRIEFING SESSIONS

One of the most important positions associated with a clinical debriefing is the role of the facilitator. For an effective debriefing to occur, it is important that the facilitator has the following skills: (a) has clinical expertise; (b) provides a supportive and safe environment for discussions; (c) has the ability to engage clinical staff members in all aspects of the discussion; (d) maintains an emphasis on teamwork processes; (e) has the ability to manage conflict and differences of opinion; and (f) ensures that the team develop solutions to clinical performance problems. Often the clinical event debriefing can be challenging since the pressures of the clinical environment, the team member's performance, skill level, and experience as well as what precipitated the clinical event are all factors that need to be considered when facilitating the debriefing session.

Debriefing the DNP project facilitates the ability of the participants to be able to actualize the project and the outcomes to the project. Debriefing facilitates learner-centered feedback by the application of reflection, self-reflection, and discovery through Kolb's (1984) phases of "converging and accommodation." The actualization of the project is a focus of learning, and this becomes concentrated on the actual events. The debriefing will enhance retention of discovered ideas.

Elements of debriefing models focus on how you felt about the situation, analysis of what was implemented well, analysis of what areas of improvement are needed, reflection on the application of the project, and what can be improved and then a summarization of the main takeaway points. This is actualized through feedback during the debriefing, which provides information to the team with intent of change and implementation. The key factor in this type of debriefing allows the team reflection to collaborate on the issues and formulate an improvement design

A debriefing facilitator can use different types of structure and incorporate a flexible learning environment centered on outcomes related to the incident and discussion that may enhance additional outcomes of the situation. In contrast, an instructor is focused on providing an infrastructure on how the project is done and not focused on analysis. More importantly, the facilitator role creates a safe debriefing environment for all participants. Ground rules are established, and the focus remains on the primary goals and objectives of the meeting and the project. The facilitator engages in active listening and will not embrace bias but suspends individual opinions. The facilitator will also clarify discussion points and enhance the discussion by asking open-ended questions. It is the facilitation of the debriefing that the participants will take action based on the knowledge and assumptions discussed during the debriefing session. Through this phase, the facilitator will create a context for learning that applies successful learning styles to all participants.

Facilitating a debriefing project requires the key stakeholders to champion the project and ensure the creation of a safe environment. Developing facilitators is key in the success of the program. Building the program will focus on identifying key opportunities to debrief, incorporating an interdisciplinary team concept with communication, education, system improvements, quality, safety, and gap closure in mind. A key focus of the facilitator is to ensure the empowerment of the participants to influence change. Once the DNP student identifies the vision of what the concept should look like, he or she should be clear about the goals and map the identified areas for implementation and improvement. Build a culture of safety and celebrate the wins!

SUMMARY

This chapter assists the DNP student in the understanding of a debriefing session as well as how to apply best practices during a clinical debriefing session. Discussion about the importance of the DNP student to be fully engaged in the clinical practice setting as a leader, change agent, and facilitator for debriefings was presented. Major discussion included an understanding of learning styles that can be used for successful debriefing sessions. Examples of how to apply Miller's Competence Pyramid for assessment and principles associated with the facilitator for debriefings were presented. Finally, examples of how to apply Kolb's educational theory during a debriefing session were presented.

REFERENCES

Agency for Healthcare Research and Quality. (2019). *TeamSTEPPS Core Curriculum 2.0 Essentials Course*. Retrieved from https://www.ahrq .gov/teamstepps/instructor/essentials/index.html
American Association of Colleges of Nursing. (2015a). Doctor of Nursing Practice (DNP) Tool Kit. *The Doctor of Nursing Practice: Current Issues and Clarifying Recommendations*. Retrieved from https://www.aacnnursing .org/DNP/Tool-Kit

American Association of Colleges of Nursing. (2015b). *APRN Clinical Training Task Force Report Brief*. Retrieved from http://www.aacn.nche.edu/news/articles/2015/aprn-white-paper

Fillion, J. S., Clements, P. T., Averill, J. B., & Virgil, G. J. (2002). Talking as a primary method of peer defusing for military personnel exposed to combat trauma. *Journal of Psychosocial Nursing and Mental Health Services*, *40*(8), 40–49. doi:10.3928/0279-3695-20020901-11

Kolb, A. Y., & Kolb, D. A. (2005). Learning styles and learning spaces: Enhancing experiential learning at a higher level. *Academy of Management Learning & Education*, *4*(2), 193–212. doi:10.5465/AMLE.2005.17268566

Kolb, D. A. (1984). *Experiential learning: Experience as the source of learning and development*. Englewood Cliffs, NJ: Prentice-Hall.

McLeod, S. (2017). *Kolb's learning styles and experiential learning cycle*. Retrieved from https://www.simplypsychology.org/learning-kolb.html

Miller, G. E. (1990). The assessment of clinical skills/competence/performance. *Academic Medicine*, *65*(9), s63–s67.

Quality and Safety Education for Nurses. (2018). *Chasing zero: Winning the war on healthcare harm*. Retrieved from http://qsen.org/publications/videos/chasing-zero-winning-the-war-on-healthcare-harm

IV INTERPRETATION, DISSEMINATION OF FINDINGS, AND BEYOND

8 | INTERPRETATION OF FINDINGS AND IMPACT ON CLINICAL PRACTICE

DENISE M. KORNIEWICZ

INTRODUCTION

The goal of the DNP project is to provide the evidence associated with improving patient outcomes that will be used to deliver care and educate others in a patient population. The American Association of Colleges of Nursing (AACN, 2006) has defined these areas to include

> any form of nursing intervention that influences health care outcomes for individuals or populations, including the direct care of individual patients, management of care for individuals and populations, administration of nursing and health care organizations, and the development and implementation of health policy. (p. 2)

Therefore, any data associated with a DNP project should be related to clinical inquiry and analyzed with the clinical research question in mind. The interpretation of the data and the results would need to be tied to the overall clinical question investigated.

As part of the DNP Essentials (AACN, 2006), it is necessary for DNP graduates to be able to integrate and demonstrate their skills in the following areas:

- Demonstrate expertise related to reflective practice
- Demonstrate expertise in the area of interest
- Ability of identify methods related to independent practice inquiry

- Present the clinical evidence by evaluating and translating research findings that improve health and the quality-of-care outcomes
- Provide leadership within organizations to develop, implement, and evaluate interventions to improve patient outcomes for diverse populations
- Utilize or contribute to healthcare policies, ethics, or law that improves population-based healthcare programs

Keeping in mind the DNP Essentials (AACN, 2006), this chapter provides a step-by-step approach on how to interpret qualitative or quantitative methods used to develop clinical projects. The first section of the chapter focuses on qualitative methods and presents how to complete the analysis and interpret the clinical findings. Then we focus on quantitative methods and interpretation of findings that are important in the understanding of evidence-based practice. Finally, we provide a discussion about the impact of the results or findings on clinical practice issues that were derived from either qualitative or quantitative methods.

INTERPRETING A QUALITATIVE DNP PROJECT

The steps associated with reviewing the qualitative data for the DNP project are dependent on the type of qualitative methods that were initially proposed. However, the steps involved for the interpretation of the data may be similar. Whether one is using a grounded theory or a phenomenological method, use of a systematic approach to review the data can be completed by following the steps listed next.

Choosing the Type of Qualitative Method

The initial step in using qualitative data methods is to decide which approach (grounded theory or phenomenological) is the best fit for the project. The investigator should determine if a structured interview will be used as a guide to survey the participants or if a general open-ended interview will be used to gather information about the experiences of patients. Whatever the approach, the important point is that the investigator is consistent with the data collection process. A few examples may include face-to-face interviews, individual interviews, or group interviews. Either way, it is important to gather the participants' "thoughts" on the matter and document, record, or enter the data into a qualitative database (Zamawe, 2015) that captures the participants' responses. Again, the data collection process is determined by the method used.

Interpreting Qualitative Results

The second step requires the investigator to review the results of the data. Qualitative data seek an understanding of the phenomenon under study versus a specific answer. Interpretation of the qualitative data begins with an overall review of the responses. If grounded theory was used (Glaser & Strauss, 1999) and open-ended structured interviews were obtained, then categorization of the data begins with collating the overall participant responses from the structured interview guide. If a phenomenological (Wimpenny & Gass, 2000) approach was used, then it would be important to categorize the data according to the concepts derived from the experiences expressed by patients about the clinical event. With the use of either qualitative method, the goal is to systematically search for broad themes or categories that emerge from the data. The themes are usually commonalities that are presented by the participants and provide relationships within the data. The objective is to search for patterns or regularities in the data. Thus, depending on the methods chosen for the DNP project, the use of themes or categories remains to be the first step for understanding the qualitative results. Table 8.1 provides an example of the use of two different qualitative methods and how to develop a systematic process to review the data and develop a list of concepts or themes.

Validating Qualitative Results

The third step to qualitative data interpretation is to validate the possible themes or categories that emerged from the data. When reviewing the data for possible themes, the investigator should list common words that have been used to describe the patient's experience during his or her clinical event. Examples may include the communication received from the provider or other staff during the clinical event, description of promptness associated with pain relief, or discussion about the laboratory tests that were needed for the diagnosis. What is important during this phase is to review the data from all participants and to develop a list of themes or concepts that are similar. If using grounded theory as the approach and a structured interview, then the data should reflect similar responses from the participants. If using a phenomenological approach, then the responses from the participants may reflect experiences of the clinical event that were similar. The flowchart (Figure 8.1) demonstrates the steps associated with reviewing qualitative data for the discussion of findings for either a grounded theory or phenomenological approach. Regardless of the qualitative methodology used, the steps to review the data are similar and require the investigator to focus on clinical expertise to interpret the data.

TABLE 8.1 Qualitative Approaches: Grounded Theory Versus a Phenomenological Approach to Review and Categorize Themes Related to Quality Patient Care

Qualitative Method	How to Review Data	Example of Theme or Concept from Participants	Developed List of Concepts
Grounded theory *(use of a structured questionnaire related to quality of patient care)*	Common words that were derived from a structured open-ended interview guide Develop list of words used by participants and categorize into common themes	• Perception of quality of care • Pain control • Comfort measures • Communication	• Quality of care • Pain • Nursing measures • Effective communication by staff
Phenomenological approach *(open-ended discussion with participants about the quality of care they received during a recent clinical event)* • Descriptive • Selective • Detailed	Meaning of an experience through identification of common themes Statements essential to experience Analysis and interpretation of every sentence	• I was anxious about the care I received • I felt that my pain was not under control • I had to wait a long time for assistance when getting out of bed • I didn't feel that the doctor told me everything about my diagnosis	• Anxiety • Pain measures • Wait period for care • Confidence in doctor

Source: From Glaser, B., & Strauss, A. (1999). *The discovery of grounded theory,* Chapter 3. (pp. 45–52). London and New York: Routledge, Taylor & Francis Group; Wimpenny, P., & Gass, J. (2000). Interviewing in phenomenology and grounded theory: is there a difference? *Journal of Advanced Nursing, 31*(6), 1485–1492.

Interpreting Qualitative Data

The fourth step in the interpretation of qualitative data findings includes reviewing the major themes to validate their consistency for further analysis. This final step may require further validation (see Figure 8.1) from other clinical staff or those who have had experience working with patients with similar issues. At this time, it is important to review the initial research question and determine if the data

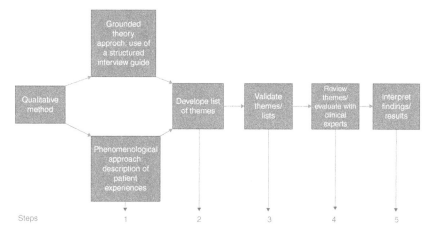

FIGURE 8.1 Steps to understand qualitative data analysis: grounded theory versus phenomenological methods.

support or confirm what was initially proposed by the investigator. It is important to have other clinical experts review the data independently and then make comparisons proposed by the investigator. This will help to further validate the overall finding of the project. Once completed, the investigator will need to reflect and discuss the themes and make any adjustments to the overall findings. Finally, a final list of themes is proposed and compared to the literature so that the results can be validated in the literature as a best-practice method. It is at this time that the investigator formulates ideas or opinions about the overall data and makes suggestions as to how the data support or negate the overall research question.

Critical Analysis of Qualitative Results

Step five includes the critical review, evaluation, synthesis, and interpretation of the qualitative data. Lincoln and Guba (1985) suggest that one way to enhance qualitative data interpretation is to evaluate the content via established criteria such as credibility, transferability, dependability, and confirmability. Lincoln and Guba (1985) further define each of these characteristics as important ways to provide rigor to the interpretation of the qualitative methodology used. Credibility refers to the truth of the findings for the participants and the believability of the findings. Inherent to establishing credibility, several techniques may be used including prolonged engagement, persistent observation, peer debriefing, triangulation, or negative case analysis. Transferability refers to demonstrating that the finding has application to other concepts. One technique for establishing transferability may reside in providing a thick or indepth description of the situation. Dependability demonstrates that the findings are consistent over time and are replicable. One technique to establish dependability would be to provide an audit of the data or a review by an individual not involved in the study. Confirmability has been defined as the accuracy of the data and reflects what the participants have stated versus the interpretation by the investigator. Other ways to establish confirmability can be by using triangulation techniques or reflexivity (Lincoln & Guba, 1985). Thus, in reviewing the list of themes developed by the investigator, it would be important to further validate against a set of specific criteria. Figure 8.2 provides an example of a matrix that can be used to evaluate a set of themes against the evaluation criteria suggested by Lincoln and Guba (1985). Upon completion of this step, the investigator can systematically review the findings with assurance that his or her interpretation of the data was valid and congruent with the methods used for the overall study.

INTERPRETING A QUANTITATIVE DNP PROJECT

The steps associated with reviewing quantitative data for the DNP project is a systematic consistent approach that can be used for reviewing any major data set. The analysis of the data set is dependent upon the initial research design that was proposed. However, the steps to interpret and present the data are similar for any quantitative project. Organizing

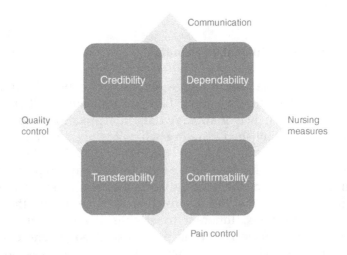

FIGURE 8.2 Matrix to systematically validate qualitative themes.

the data in a meaningful way will assist in the final interpretation of the results. Following the steps listed next will assist in the organization and final review process of a DNP quantitative project.

Quantitative Data Collection

Step one includes data collection for the project. Most DNP quantitative studies consist of survey data, evaluation of stored data (electronic health records [EHRs]), use of data from national registries, or use of quality-of-care indices that provide patient scores (Polit & Beck, 2012). Quantitative data analysis answers specific research questions posed by the investigator. It is during this phase that the investigator collects the data and enters the data into an electronic database (EPI Info, 2017; SPSS, 2017). Guidelines associated with quantitative data collection plans can be found in Box 8.1.

BOX 8.1 Review Guidelines for Quantitative Data Collection Methods

- Were the methods suggested appropriate for the research question?
- Did the investigator predetermine sample size?
- Do the instruments chosen measure the variables (quality of care) being tested?
- Were data collection procedures (data collection plan) developed for consistency?
- Was there a training period developed to train other data collectors involved in the study?
- Did the investigator oversee the data collection procedures to review any consistencies during the data collection period?
- Was the setting (number of patients, staff) appropriate for the population of study?
- How did the investigator deal with changes in clinical practice or staff during the data collection period?
- Did the investigator have to change the data collection procedures during the study period; if so, what was changed and how did it impact on the data collection?
- Who entered the data into an electronic database and were they proficient in entering the data?
- Were the data rechecked for any errors during the data input stage?

Levels of Measurement

The second step is to present the results, which include an overall description of the population studied. Data analysis tests are guided by the level of data analyzed. Depending on the level of measurement used, presentation of the findings may be displayed by using data tables or graphs that can provide a clear representation of the population of interest. What is important is that the data are categorized within the four levels of measurement: nominal, ordinal,interval, and ratio (Howlett, Rago, & Gabiola, 2014); see Table 8.2.

Descriptive data analysis includes measures of central tendency (mean, median, and mode) and variation (range and standard deviation); see Howlett et al. (2014). The dependent and independent variables of the study will need to be further explored in relation to the mean, median, and mode. Analysis of these data will provide an overall description of the participants' characteristics and numeric presentation of the data for visualization. Examples of description data may include the demographics associated with the study group such as age, income,

TABLE 8.2 Quantitative Levels of Measurement, Definition, Example, and Statistical Measure

Levels of Measurement	Definition	Example
Nominal	Differentiates between subjects based on categories.	Groups data according to name, gender, or age.
Ordinal	Compares levels of data to each other.	Comparisons between values such as sick versus healthy, independent versus dependent. Use of percentages can be obtained.
Interval	Measures differences between points.	Example such as a yardstick that measures inches, feet (range between 1 and 36 inches). Use of average is possible.
Ratio	Measures data points that are standardized and meaningful. Must have a *true zero* to be considered ratio data.	Examples include height (measures in centimeters) or weight (scale).

TABLE 8.3 Presentation of Quantitative Data for Demographic Data

Variable	n	%	Total
Age			
Men	7 (55–71)	35	
Women	13 (51–86)	65	
			20
Gender			
Male	6	30	
Female	13	65	
Transgender	1	.05	
Other	0		100
Race			
American Indian or	1	.05	
Alaska Native	0		
Asian	2	10	
Black or African	9	45	
American Native	0		
Hawaiian			
Other Pacific	0		
Islander			
White	8	40	
			100

sexual orientation, ethnicity, and other variables initially described in the proposal. An example of how to present the demographics of a quantitative study can be found in Table 8.3.

Validity and Reliability

Quantitative studies are designed to measure variables that can be expressed in a numeric fashion. Any instrument that is used to measure a variable such as the quality of patient care should be reliable, valid, and provide the psychometrics associated with sensitivity and specificity (Sullivan, 2011). Reliability of an instrument refers to the consistency that it measures the targeted variable. For example, a survey associated with the quality of patient care and the scores used to test "quality of care" would need to have been reported several times by different groups of patients. Reliability refers to the stability, internal consistency, and equivalence of the instrument that has been used over time (Sullivan, 2011). Reliability scores of an instrument should have been reported in the literature and become important as a comparison criterion for selection of an instrument.

Validity of an instrument simply means that the instrument measures what it is supposed to measure. Validity refers to different aspects of the instrument such as face, content, and construct validity (Polit & Beck, 2012). During this third step, the investigator will need to describe the instrument used to measure the variable of interest (quality of patient care) and provide the data associated with the reliability and validity of the instrument used for the project. Once completed, the investigator will be able to compare the results of his or her study against the results of others who have used the same instrument. This provides an opportunity for the investigator to begin to analyze the data and reflect on the meaning of his or her results as compared to what has been previously published.

Quantitative Data Analysis

The fourth step in the review of quantitative DNP projects includes the analysis of data. Analysis of the quantitative data project requires the use of inferential statistical methods and is dependent upon the initial methods described in the DNP proposal. Inferential statistics are based on the law of probability and allows the investigator to make inferences about the data collected (Kern, 2014). Inferential statistics include discussion about the distribution of the population or sample, estimates associated with the standard error of the mean, and an understanding of the range of values or confidence intervals (Kern, 2014). Since there are a variety of inferential statistical methods available, what is important is that the analysis is consistent with answering the initial clinical research question. Often quantitative analysis measures relationships that exist between research variables. Use of inferential statistics requires that the investigator has reviewed the general data output from the data set and has systematically reviewed the overall data for any errors (type I or type II) associated with data analysis (Kern, 2014).

Further statistical methods may be applied, depending on the overall clinical question, especially if the investigator proposed a specific analysis in the methods portion of the DNP proposal. Nonparametric versus parametric statistics can be used for the analysis of the results. Thus, a basic understanding of the use of various statistical measures will aid in the overall analysis of the results.

Quantitative Data Presentation

The final step in reviewing a quantitative DNP project is the presentation of the data. Once the analysis is completed, the investigator will need to group the data in a systematic manner. Often the descriptive statistics include the frequencies of the participant responses for each of the demographic items. Other tables summarizing survey responses may be used to show the overall findings related to the clinical question. Creating visuals of the data assists the reader in the understanding of the overall findings of the project. Finally, the most important aspect of the presentation of the findings is to present the "need to know data" versus showing all the data derived from the computerized analysis (SPSS). The need to know data refers to the findings that specifically answer the clinical research question. If there are other findings derived from the data analysis, then the data should be deferred to be presented at a later time. It is important that the investigator focuses the DNP findings specifically on answering the initial clinical question.

Mixed Methods: Qualitative and Quantitative

The term "mixed methods" refers to the use of both quantitative and qualitative research methods. This research methodology requires a systematic integration of utilizing data without doing separate data collection or analysis processes. Mixing refers to the process whereby the qualitative and quantitative elements are interlinked to produce a fuller account of the research problem (Glogowska, 2011; Zhang & Creswell, 2013). This integration can occur at any stage(s) of the research process but is vital to the rigor of the mixed methods research (Glogowska, 2011).

Mixed methods research has been used in the social sciences and has now been expanded into the health and medical sciences including nursing, family medicine, social work, mental health, pharmacy, allied health, and others (Creswell, 2014). Depending on the research question, mixed methods provide an avenue for increased communication across disciplines and benefit patient care associated with functional status and activities of daily living. Mixed methods studies assist practitioners in how to apply best practices related to the outcomes of patient care, cost, quality, and patient experiences.

The research design of a mixed methods research study requires that the methodological approaches ensure that the rigor of the design supports the research question(s) of the study. In planning a mixed methods design, consider the following: (a) create a rationale for using mixed methods; (b) investigate the philosophical approach of the study; (c) identify the various mixed methods designs; (d) determine the required skills needed to complete the project; (e) understand the project management of the study; (f) justify the integration of both the qualitative and quantitative aspects of the study; and (g) ensure that rigor is demonstrated in the analysis of the project (Zhang & Creswell,

2013). Although the use of a mixed methods design requires additional upfront development, there are several positive outcomes that must be considered by healthcare practitioners. These include: (a) comparison of quantitative and qualitative data that may assist in the understanding of any patient care contradictions; (b) provides participant's point of view and ensures that the participant has a voice; (c) cultivates scholarly interaction among multidisciplinary healthcare teams; (d) enhances methodological flexibility; and (e) provides more comprehensive data through the integration of data and analysis of the research question(s). On the other hand, there are some disadvantages that have been reported in the literature (Walsh & Evans, 2014). These include: (a) increased complexity of implementing the research project since data collection methods and analysis may be difficult because of timing sample size limitations; (b) use of a multidisciplinary team may require increased sample size and increased discussion periods so that all data and analysis include input from all members of the team; and (c) mixed methods studies may require more resources due to the increased manpower needed to collect data and complete analysis and discussion of all findings (Scammon et al., 2013).

IMPACT OF THE CLINICAL FINDINGS

Regardless of the research design or methods used to frame the DNP project, the final step in the interpretation of the results specifically focuses on the impact that the data will have on clinical practice (Figure 8.3) and contribution to evidence-based clinical outcomes.

Discussion of what impact the findings may have on clinical practice can be framed by answering the following questions:

- What impact, if any, did the project have on clinical practice?
- Did the findings support the investigator's initial "hunch" about the clinical question?
- Did the findings describe the similarities or differences found in the literature?
- Were the findings new?
- What implications, if any, do the findings have on education or clinical practice?
- What implications, if any, do the findings have on improving clinical practice guidelines?

This final step includes thoroughly interpreting the results and developing recommendations to generate or change current

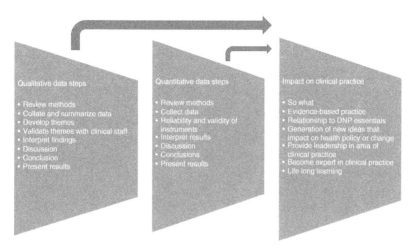

FIGURE 8.3 Qualitative or quantitative methods and impact on clinical practice.

evidence-based clinical practice. The conclusions drawn from the study will need to reflect content that was consistent with the initial clinical question or phenomenon of study. The interpretation of the data and their impact on clinical practice should systematically be presented in a manner that reflects evidence-based clinical inquiry. A few general principles that may be used to guide the investigator to further develop clinical inquiry related to the findings may include answers to "so what" questions prior to writing the results. Examples of the "so what" questions may include:

- So what do your results mean when evaluating against current clinical practice trends?
- So, what do the data mean?
- What impact do these findings have on clinical practice?
- Do the data provide paths for future research?
- Do the data answer the initial clinical question posed?
- Do the data influence the development of health policy (local, regional, or national)?
- Do the data influence how healthcare is delivered or improve current health delivery systems?
- Can conclusions provide additional evidence about the proposed clinical inquiry?

Further, interpretation of the findings requires the investigator to be knowledgeable about the content area of study and to articulate the similarities and differences associated with the findings. A critical evaluation of the findings provides for the enhancement of evidence-based clinical practice. Discussion about what worked and what did not work will need to be provided in the findings. Critically evaluating the findings may provide the groundwork for clinical practice changes and suggest improvements for quality patient care. Thus, it is important for the investigator to provide the rationale as to how the findings have been supported or not supported in the clinical research. New findings from the project need to be highlighted in the discussion to reflect their importance and to suggest changes related to clinical practice.

It is important to keep in mind the DNP Essentials (AACN, 2006) when reviewing the final findings, discussion, and conclusions of the DNP project. For example, reviewing the results and championing the use of reflective practice provides a framework for thinking about the findings and how they impact clinical practice. This includes individual and collective reflection, action, and transformative learning that supports the further development of clinical inquiry (Johns, 2005). Reflective practice may include discussions about how to revise a clinical procedure or experience or changing social norms related to values that impact on changing practice. One example, using the concepts of reflective practice, was the changes that occurred as a result of understanding the transmission of HIV. As a result of clinical research and the further understanding about the transmission and treatment of HIV, healthcare policies were changed and clinical guidelines were instituted. Evaluating the structures, processes, and outcomes related to the DNP project provides a model to reflect and think about how the clinical project may transform clinical practice. Therefore, the use of reflection as a way to have a deeper understanding of the clinical results may assist in providing changes to real-life clinical situations.

The second DNP Essential (AACN, 2006) includes the ability to demonstrate expertise in the area of clinical practice. The findings, conclusions, and discussion about new and ongoing clinical changes related to the clinical question would be one way to demonstrate further clinical knowledge expertise. The investigator's ability to provide the reader with an understanding of his or her expanded clinical knowledge related to evidence-based practice and futuristic clinical practice changes may be another way to demonstrate advanced practice expertise. Additional examples may include the development of new clinical standards related to the specific clinical question or the development of local or national clinical guidelines for a specific patient population.

Keeping in mind the other DNP Essentials (AACN, 2006) that are related to independent practice, the translation of research findings to improve the quality of care and discussion about improving healthcare guidelines may be areas to highlight in the final DNP project. Whatever the clinical topic chosen, the importance of generating new ideas that enhance current clinical guidelines to promote safe healthcare should be included in the overall discussion. Finally, the competencies that are recommended by the AACN (2006) Essentials will need to be discussed in relation to leadership skills and the utilization of healthcare policies that may improve patient outcomes

Finally, the interpretation of the data and their impact on clinical practice is one of the most important aspects of the DNP project. In fact, it is the future graduates of the DNP programs who will assist in changing clinical care and providing clinical outcomes that may influence change for the advancement of clinical practice. Concepts associated with changing current clinical practice, modifying patient treatment for better patient outcomes, suggesting changes associated with the delivery of healthcare, and developing health policies are all examples that may result from a DNP project. Therefore, the interpretation of the findings and conclusions of the DNP project need to be presented to other healthcare providers to further the science of evidence-based practice.

SUMMARY

This chapter focused on the use of qualitative, quantitative, or mixed methods research designs that can be used to investigate DNP clinical projects. Content associated with choosing the right research method, data collection, and interpretation of results was presented. Discussion about the impact of the results and how the results will impact on clinical practice was presented. Key concepts associated with data analysis and the importance of how to interpret the results based on the impact data have on evidence-based practice were discussed. The essential components associated with the presentation of data and understanding how to use data for their meaning in clinical practice were provided.

APPLICATION EXERCISES: QUANTITATIVE VERSUS QUALITATIVE DATA METHODS

Introduction

The use of quantitative versus qualitative data methods is important when designing healthcare research topics. Often, researchers tend to prefer one method over the other. However, the use of mixed methods research for a single study has begun to emerge. There is evidence in the literature that mixed methods are being critically appraised to assist in the understanding of theory, design, and use as an approach to successfully generate insights into complex research questions (Van den Bruel, Jones, Thompson, & Mant, 2016). However, the integration of the data must be clearly applied at the outset of the study. Therefore, it is important for the clinician to understand the differences in the application of the research methods.

The major components of a well-designed mixed methods research study include the following:

- Collecting and analyzing both quantitative (closed-ended) and qualitative (open-ended) data such as interviews, general health, and well-being surveys
- Using data collection procedures to analyze data appropriate to each method's tradition such as appropriate sample size for data analysis
- Integrating the data during data collection, analysis, or discussion
- Using data procedures that implement qualitative or quantitative components with the same sample or with different samples. To review your skills at understanding the differences between quantitative and qualitative methods, take the simple 10-item quiz in Box 8.2. Answers for the quiz can be found in Chapter 11, Application Exercise Answer Keys

Using Qualitative Research Methods

Qualitative research methods explore a particular phenomenon. In nursing and healthcare, the use of qualitative methods has described patient experiences with illness, changes in lifestyle, activities of daily living, or any experience related to their well-being. There are a variety of qualitative methods that can be used such as grounded theory, phenomenology, ethnography, and qualitative descriptive methods (Strauss & Corbin, 1998). No matter which method is followed, the researcher chooses the assumptions and purposes, and the method is based on the overall research question. For example, if a researcher is interested in understanding the process involved in the occurrence of a phenomenon, the researcher would choose grounded theory. However, if the researcher is interested in the meaning of the phenomenon of study, then he or she would utilize phenomenology. Regardless of the method, data are collected as interviews, observation, or document/photo review. The

BOX 8.2 Exercise 1: 10-Item Quiz: Quantitative Versus Qualitative Methods*

1. Using a written questionnaire with closed-ended questions (e.g., Yes/No) to survey a large number of gunshot victims who may be experiencing posttraumatic stress disorder.
   a. Qualitative research
   b. Quantitative research
   c. Both
2. Observing the effects of using a treat such as candy when teaching a kindergarten child to keep quiet on command.
   a. Qualitative research
   b. Quantitative research
   c. Both
3. Conducting an experiment to investigate whether having regular rest breaks during exercise sessions improves overall physical performance.
   a. Qualitative research
   b. Quantitative research
   c. Both
4. Investigating ways in which women are portrayed in the print media of medical journals by analyzing advertisements.
   a. Qualitative research
   b. Quantitative research
   c. Both
5. Observing whether physicians conform to general practice guidelines by counting the number of physicians who disobey electronic record sign-ins during medical rounds.
   a. Qualitative research
   b. Quantitative research
   c. Both
6. Observing the social interactions of nurses in an intensive care area by using predetermined items on an observation checklist.
   a. Qualitative research
   b. Quantitative research
   c. Both
7. Organizing a small number of participants into a discussion group to study racial discrimination in the workplace.
   a. Qualitative research
   b. Quantitative research
   c. Both

(*continued*)

BOX 8.2 Exercise 1: 10-Item Quiz: Quantitative Versus Qualitative
Methods* (*continued*)

---

8. Testing the relationship between the scores on an intelligence
   test and scores on a personality test.
   a. Qualitative research
   b. Quantitative research
   c. Both
9. Studying the behavior of newborn infants by observing and
   recording their second-by-second movements during their first
   72 hours of life following birth.
   a. Qualitative research
   b. Quantitative research
   c. Both
10. Investigating the effects of observing violence by analyzing
    and interpreting children's drawings after they have watched
    violent cartoons on television.
    a. Qualitative research
    b. Quantitative research
    c. Both

---

*A score of 70% or greater indicates that you have a good understanding of the
differences between quantitative and qualitative data methods.

overall objective of qualitative research is not the accumulation of information; rather, it is gaining an understanding about the phenomenon
of study.

In order to apply a qualitative method, the following exemplar
will use a grounded theory approach to understand the concept of pain
with cancer patients.

Mrs. Smith is a 62-year-old woman who has been a patient for many
years. For the past few months, she has complained of increasingly
severe upper abdominal pain and weight loss. An ultrasound
ordered by Dr. Minor revealed a mass highly suspicious for primary liver cancer. As the disease progresses, Mrs. Smith is increasingly in more pain. At night, she cries when she thinks no one can
hear her. In the morning, she is silent again—and she has not spoken more than a few words to her daughters in several days since
her last talk with Chaplain Olsen. She told the chaplain that she
wanted a drug or treatment that would not make her feel anything
at all. One day, Mrs. Smith and her three daughters ask Dr. Minor

for help. The two older daughters want to abide by their mother's wishes and help her, in her words, "sleep through the whole process," as much as possible. Gloria, her youngest daughter, wants her mother to have pain care, but wants her to be conscious so that they can talk with one another.

As a home care nurse, you contact Dr. Minor to report Mrs. Smith's right upper quadrant abdominal pain, rated 10/10 and described as sharp, pressing, pulling, spreading, drawing, tight, nauseating, fearful, unbearable, and dreadful that is not controlled with 200 mg oral morphine taken every 3 to 4 hours. Mrs. Smith has been taking 900 mg oral morphine every 3 hours and indomethacin 25 mg orally every 6 hours. Dr. Minor asks you for a recommendation about what to try next to help Mrs. Smith to get pain relief.

Exercise 2: Focused Interview Guide

Using pain as the concept of study, develop a *focused interview guide* that would be used to understand the patient's experience about pain. It is important to think about the variables associated with the individual's personal experience of pain, age, gender, cause of pain, diagnosis, sensory or emotional experience of pain, when developing a focused interview guide. Remember, focused interview guides are developed for conversations with the patient in order to ascertain specific aspects about the phenomenon of study, in this case "pain." The answer for Exercise 2 can be found in Chapter 11, Application Exercise Answer Keys.

Using Quantitative Research Methods

Quantitative research methods are a systematic approach investigating research questions in which numerical data are collected. It involves describing a situation or event that answers specific questions by measuring or counting. A quantitative approach is concerned with finding evidence that either supports or contradicts an idea or hypothesis that is postulated. A hypothesis is a statement that predicts an answer such as whether increasing clinical hours to nurse training will provide more proficient clinical nursing outcomes.

Much like qualitative data, quantitative data can be gathered from a variety of sources such as questionnaires, interviews, observation, transaction logs, or surveys (Creswell, 2014). Depending on the type of data a researcher is collecting, what is significant is that once all data are collected, it is important to organize, summarize, and do exploratory data analysis. This can be communicated in the form of tables, graphic displays, or summary statistics. Additionally, quantitative data can be analyzed for similarities, differences, or relationships among or between data variables.

There are advantages and disadvantages when using quantitative methods. The advantages include: (a) ability to obtain large numbers in a study, (b) allows for a broader study, (c) enhances for generalization of results, (d) uses prescribed procedures to ensure reliability and validity of measures used in the study, (e) research can be replicated, compared to similar studies and can facilitate comparisons across categories, and (f) avoids researcher bias since researchers keep a distance from participants in the study. The disadvantages include: (a) data collection can be narrow and sometimes superficial, (b) results may provide less elaborate accounts of human perception, (c) may lack "real-world" results since the environment may be readily controlled, such as in a laboratory, (d) preset answers may not reflect how participants really feel about the subject matter, and (e) the development of standard questions by a research investigator can lead to bias and false representation. Regardless of the advantages and disadvantages associated with the use of quantitative research, most research investigators prefer to review the evidence available about the study topic and decide which research methodology best fits their research question. In order to begin to interpret research manuscripts associated with quantitative research projects, it is best to follow a systematic research critique to comprehensively evaluate if the research design was appropriate for the study.

Exercise 3. Critique of a Quantitative Research Project

One of the most important skills needed to evaluate quantitative research studies is the ability to determine if the research methods used were able to answer the posed research question. The following guidelines provide a process to determine if the quantitative research study answered the research question.

- Does the research question imply a relationship between the independent and dependent variables?
- Is the research question clearly stated?
- Is there an intervention or treatment suggested?
- What type of research design was described?
- Are the methods clearly described (e.g., sample, procedures for the study, treatment or nontreatment groups)?

- What types of comparisons are made and do these comparisons provide support for the independent and dependent variables of the study?
- Were the data collection procedures described?
- Was the data collected appropriate for the study?

Using a guide to evaluate a quantitative research study will assist in determining if a study would be able to be replicated and provide new knowledge for clinical practice.

Access the following website: jcm.asm.org/content/jcm/28/4/787 .full.pdf. Using the research critique guide provided, critique this journal article to evaluate the quantitative measure used.

REFERENCES

American Association of Colleges of Nursing. (2006). *DNP essentials.* Retrieved from http://www.aacnnursing.org/Education-Resources/ AACN-Essentials

Creswell, J. W. (2014). *Research design: Qualitative, quantitative, and mixed methods approaches.* Thousand Oaks, CA: Sage Publications.

Epi Info. (2017). Division of Health Informatics & Surveillance (DHIS), Center for Surveillance, Epidemiology and Laboratory Services (CSELS). Retrieved from https://www.cdc.gov/ophss/csels/index.html

Glaser, B., & Strauss, A. (1999). *The discovery of grounded theory* (pp. 45–52). London and New York: Routledge, Taylor & Francis Group.

Glogowska, M. (2011). Paradigms, pragmatism and possibilities: Mixed-methods research in speech and language therapy. *International Journal of Language Communication Disorders, 46,* 251–260. doi:10.3109/13682822.2010.507614

Howlett, B., Rago, E., & Gabiola, T. (2014). *Foundations of evidence-based practice* (pp. 31–52). Burlington, MA: Jones and Bartlett.

Johns, C. (2005). Expanding the gates of perception. In C. Johns & D. Freshwater (Eds.), *Transforming nursing through reflective practice* (2nd ed., pp. 1–12). Oxford, UK: Blackwell Science.

Kern, S. (2014). *Inferential statistics, power estimates, and study design formalities continue to suppress biomedical innovation.* Baltimore, MD: The Sidney Kimmel Comprehensive Cancer Center at Johns Hopkins, Department of Oncology. Retrieved from http://pathology.jhu.edu/department/ research/monograph.cfm

Lincoln, Y. S., & Guba, E. G. (1985). *Naturalistic inquiry.* Newbury Park, CA: Sage Publications.

Mathews, K., Phelan, J., Jones, N. A., Konya, S., Marks, R., Pratt, B. M., . . . Bentley, M. (2017). *2015 National Content Test Race and Ethnicity Analysis Report.* Retrieved from https://www2.census.gov/programs-surveys/ decennial/2020/program-management/final-analysis-reports/ 2015nct-race-ethnicity-analysis.pdf

Polit, D., & Beck, C. (2012). *Nursing research: Generating and assessing evidence for nursing practice* (9th ed.). Philadelphia, PA: Lippincott Williams & Wilkins.

Scammon, D. L., Tomoaia-Cotisel, A., Day, R. L., Day, J., Kim, J., Waitzman, N. J., . . . Magill, M. K. (2013). Connecting the dots and merging meaning: Using mixed methods to study primary care delivery transformation. *Health Services Research, 48*, 2181–2207. doi:10.1111/1475-6773.12114

SPSS. (2017). *Statistical software*. Retrieved from http://www.spss.com.hk/software/statistics

Strauss, A., & Corbin, J. (1998). *Basic qualitative research* (2nd ed.). Thousand Oaks, CA: Sage Publications.

Sullivan, G. M. (2011). A primer on the validity of assessment instruments. *Journal of Graduate Medical Education, 3*(2), 119–120. doi:10.4300/JGME-D-11-00075.1

Van den Bruel, A., Jones, C., Thompson, M., & Mant, D. (2016). C-reactive protein point-of-care testing in acutely ill children: A mixed methods study in primary care. *Archives of Disease in Childhood, 10*, 1136.

Walsh, D., & Evans, K. (2014). Critical realism: An important theoretical perspective for midwifery research. *Midwifery, 30*, e1–e6. doi:10.1016/j.midw.2013.09.002

Wimpenny, P., & Gass, J. (2000). Interviewing in phenomenology and grounded theory: Is there a difference? *Journal of Advanced Nursing, 31*(6), 1485–1492. doi:10.1097/MLR.0b013e31824642fd

Zamawe, F. C. (2015). The implication of using NVivo Software in qualitative data analysis: Evidence-based reflections. *Malawi Medical Journal, 27*(1), 13–15. doi:10.4314/mmj.v27i1.4

Zhang, W., & Creswell, J. (2013). The use of "mixing" procedure of mixed methods in health services research. *Medical Care, 51*, e51–e57. doi:10.1097/MLR.0b013e31824642fd

DISSEMINATION OF FINDINGS, PRESENTATIONS, AND PUBLICATIONS

CAROL PATTON

INTRODUCTION

The *Essentials of Doctoral Education for Advanced Nursing Practice* (American Association of Colleges of Nursing [AACN], 2006), Essential III: Clinical Scholarship and Analytical Methods for Evidence-Based Practice focuses on scholarship and research as hallmarks of doctoral education. The DNP project provides an excellent beginning to disseminate findings, presentations, and publishing and to begin a trajectory of clinical scholarship. Brown and Crabtree (2013) suggest that DNPs are expected to disseminate scholarly works through professional conferences, peer-reviewed articles, and presentation at local, regional, and national meetings.

One of the most familiar models of scholarship was developed by Earnest Boyer (1997). Boyer's Model of Scholarship focuses on four components of scholarly engagement including discovery, integration, application, and teaching (Table 9.1).

DNP students are prepared in their DNP programs to meet each of the DNP Essentials including Essential III, which focuses on *Clinical Scholarship and Analytical Methods for Evidence-Based Practice* (AACN, 2006).

The focus of this chapter is on strategies to assist the DNP student to understand how to disseminate scholarship in a variety of ways. For example, there is emphasis on how to present material via oral or written presentations to local, regional, and national constituents at annual conferences. The importance of formatting, adhering to presentation, and following author guidelines ispresented. Additionally, content

TABLE 9.1 Boyer's Model for DNP Scholarship

Components/ Type of Boyer's Model of Scholarship	Purpose of the Components/Type of Boyer's Model of Scholarship	Evidence That the Purpose of the Components/Type of Boyer's Model of Scholarship Is Met
1. Discovery	Creation and/or assimilation of new knowledge through systematic reviews of the literature or a meta-analysis of the existing body of science and evidence	Publishing and presenting in peer-reviewed venues. Write and publish a systematic review. Write and publish a meta-analysis. Give a podium presentation or a poster presentation at a national meeting.
2. Integration	Interpreting and integrating knowledge and translating science into practice	Write about the experience and process of interpreting and integrating knowledge and translating science into practice. Write about one's personal or professional experience in the role of the DNP-prepared nurse as a change agent in interpreting and integrating knowledge and translating science into practice.
3. Application	Applying scientific knowledge and best practice to address nursing and healthcare issues in a global society	Identify and write about how the DNP-prepared nurse can create sustainable change in the U.S. healthcare system through practice change, being an executive nurse leader, and the role of the DNP-prepared nurse as a policy developer or reformer to improve health status of individuals, families, groups, aggregates of patients or populations.
4. Teaching	Teaching individuals, families, groups, aggregates of patients or populations based on the scientific knowledge available in contemporary science and literature	Write about the processes and science behind successful teaching strategies and best practice to improve patient outcomes. Use scientific evidence and best practice to create sustainable health behavior change and improve health status of individuals, families, groups, aggregates of patients or populations.

Source: Adapted from Boyer, E. L. (1997). *Scholarship reconsidered: Priorities of the professoriate.* San Francisco, CA: Jossey-Bass.

includes concepts related to peer review of a manuscript or presentation, authorship, and contributions by other committee members or peers. A discussion about the best way to present and disseminate one's DNP project findings as a scholar is provided.

DETERMINING AUTHORSHIP

Sometimes it is efficacious and helpful to present or write as a team or a small group. For example, one team member may be a content expert while another peer, coworker, or faculty member has the knowledge, skills, and competencies to write or present the project or help prepare a paper or poster presentation. In these cases, it is essential to determine the order of authorship prior to completing the scholarly endeavor.

There are several factors associated with the development of a scholarly undertaking whether it is a presentation or a publication. It is important to determine first, second, or third authorship so that each person is ranked in order of the contributions made during the conception and completion of the project. The first author is usually the person who completed the project and his or her responsibilities include providing the other authors with the first to last drafts of the manuscript or project. The second and third authors are individuals who have contributed their expertise such as statistical or clinical input and have written components of the manuscript. Faculty members who have substantially assisted in the development of a manuscript and have edited or rewritten it for publication are usually placed as the last author of the project. The "last position" often denotes mentorship of the first author. The position one holds as an author is essential and should be completed at the outset of the project or manuscript.

Professional committees and publishers are very clear that every author whose name is on the scholarly work must have made a substantive and significant contribution to the scholarly work. Scholarly works such as scientific manuscripts stand the risk of being rescinded if there are authors added to the work who did not make a substantive contribution to the work. It is unacceptable to put someone's name as an author on an article if that person made little to no contribution.

PRESENTATION OF ORAL OR POSTER PROJECTS

The manner in which the DNP student will present material via oral or written presentation to local, regional, and national constituents depends on several variables. The focus of the DNP student's project and scholarship determines which venues or opportunities the DNP student pursues. For example, conferences and professional meetings depend on nurses to disseminate and share their scholarly work to key stakeholders. Typically, key stakeholders attending local, regional, and national constituents have similar interests or are from a like group of stakeholders. There are numerous professional nursing organizations that may be interested in the DNP student's scholarship since they want to learn how the DNP student's work can be translated into their practice setting or change their nursing leadership style. The important point is that there is a "good fit" between the scholarly work and the professional event requesting a "call for abstract." The key is to decide where you want to present and the topics that are published by the different professional organizations. Each conference or journal will usually have a theme and specific objectives. Check to see if the theme is relevant to the DNP project and that the topic is aligned with the conference themes.

Oral papers or poster presentations usually occur 1 year prior to the actual meeting date. Both oral and poster sessions require an abstract submission; however, a poster presentation requires submission of a poster. An example of an accepted poster session has been provided in Exhibit 9.1.

If accepted for either a poster or an oral presentation, it is essential to be available to attend.

EXHIBIT 9.1 A Poster Session: "Integrating Social Determinants of Health Into Doctoral Nursing Curriculum: Best Practice for an Innovative 21st Century Nursing Curriculum"

Dr. Carol Patton
Drexel University College of Nursing and Health Professions

Introduction

- There is a paradigm shift occurring in U.S. healthcare delivery and health policy, and the United States can no longer afford to pay for chronic care at the rate it has for the past 40 years.
- There is a clear and compelling need in the United States to have a healthcare paradigm shift from illness care to a focus on primary, secondary, and tertiary prevention.

(continued)

- Doctoral nursing curriculum must prepare DNP practitioners and nurse leaders who are creative and innovative in 21st century healthcare organizations focusing on primary, secondary, and tertiary prevention as models of care.
- The impetus for change in the U.S. paradigm of care must be on not only primary, secondary, and tertiary prevention, but the focus must shift from individual patient care to "population-focused" care.

Purpose

The focus of this presentation is to:

1. Examine best practice and strategies integrating social determinants of health into doctoral nursing curriculum.
2. Increase awareness and sensitivity of the present and future role of the DNP in leading health innovations in 21st century healthcare organizations.
3. Examine the outcome/impact of DNP-led initiatives in 21st century healthcare organizations as a result of population-focused healthcare.
4. Identify key factors of a healthcare paradigm that integrates the three levels of prevention (primary, secondary, and tertiary prevention) and "population-focused" care.

What Is "Population Health"?

- A population focuses on a group of people in a specified geographic region.
- Population health can be examined by several characteristics.
- Population health is "multidimensional."
- The CDC vital statistics can help us examine our populations and characteristics, knowing where and how to integrate health promotion initiatives.
- When teaching population health, we must teach students about social determinants of health.

(continued)

How Do We Fit One More Concept or Topic Into Our Existing DNP Curriculum?

- We must critically assess our curriculum for how and where to integrate social determinants of health into the courses without necessarily creating a new course.
- Examine and assess the AACN DNP Essentials and where best to fit content and learning for social determinants of health.

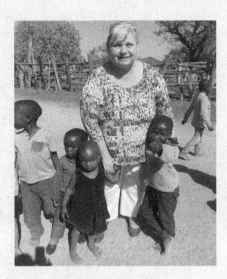

History of Disease Prevention!

- As long ago as 2500 AD, Hippocrates spoke about a physician's pledge to "keep patients from harm and the need to understand the influence of external sickness and disease."
- Much of the longevity and healthy outcomes we are experiencing are related to health promotion and disease prevention.
- *Healthy People 2020* goals have made a huge impact on health outcomes for U.S. populations, particularly our vulnerable populations.
- The time has come in the United States tot shift health policy to health promotion for populations. However, there are many strong underpinnings for how we achieve these goals related to social determinants of health.

(*continued*)

- As a nation and as healthcare professionals, nurses must be creators and innovators to foster and promote healthcare initiatives and policy that examine and take into account social determinants of health.
- Doctoral nursing programs must integrate essential content and clinical competencies that foster and promote social determinants of health grounded in all populations.

Critical Questions to Ask to Assess and Where to Place Social Determinants of Health in the DNP Curriculum

Social Determinants of Health

- One's physical and social environment including culture and climate plays a role in health outcomes and disease.
- Into which courses do these concepts best fit?
- Does your DNP curriculum need a complete course or program revision or slight assignment modification?
- What kinds of learning activities and exercises will enhance student learning and application of the concepts of social determinants of health?

References and Linkages Between Social Determinants of Health and Health Outcomes

Global Social Determinants of Health
http://www.who.int/evidence/forum/EVIPNetSDH
weekInterview.pdf

Improving Population Health
http://www.improvingpopulationhealth.org/blog/
what-are-health-factorsdeterminants.html

Social Determinants of Health: Healthy People 2020
https://www.healthypeople.gov/2020/topics-objectives/topic/
social-determinants-of-health

Developing Learning Activities and Assignments That Link Social Determinants of Health to Health Outcomes

- Expose DNP students to learning activities and assignments linked to databases in their state or community to see how one small proj.ect can change social determinants and population-focused outcomes

(continued)

- Integrate social determinants of health to health outcomes and examine strategies for students to measure their health promotion interventions in valid and reliable ways.
- Encourage DNP students to design and implement capstone or final projects that include and influence social determinants of health for populations.
- May want to link social determinants of health to health policy or population-focused initiatives in the local, regional, state, national, or international level.

Suggested Epidemiology and Population Health Concepts to Integrate Into the DNP Curriculum

- Epidemiologic perspectives and determinants of health
- Settings for health promotion
- Communication technology and health promotion
- Models of health behavior
- Genetics and genomics

AACN, American Association of Colleges of Nursing; CDC, Centers for Disease Control and Prevention.

There are a variety of ways to locate a "call for abstracts." For example, peer-reviewed, scholarly journals have a section announcing upcoming conferences and contact information. Professional organizations also email their membership regarding the "call for abstracts" and provide follow-up emails as to the due date when final submissions are scheduled. Some conferences will even ask about availability for specific days during the conference as the date and time of the oral paper or poster presentation will often not be decided until after all abstracts have been submitted and accepted for presentation.

While the DNP student may be familiar with conferences or peer-reviewed, professional journals explicit to one's current role, DNP faculty mentors and project chairs often have ideas about conferences that would be a good fit with the focus of the DNP project. The "call for abstracts" clearly identifies the conference objectives and provides detail and specificity on requirements for the submission. For example, the "call for abstracts" describes in detail what is needed, where to submit, and due date. The guidelines for the "call for abstracts" must be explicitly followed since it provides the key components for a "call for abstracts" (Table 9.2).

TABLE 9.2 Key Components for a "Call for Abstracts"

Key Component	Description	Example
Conference Title, Location, and Dates	Provides key information regarding the specific conference	*Philippine Nurses Association of America, Inc. Second Global Summit of Filipino Nurses 20XX and the 11th International Nursing Conference January 25 and 26, 20XX ◆ Blue Leaf Filipinas, Manila, Philippines*
Call for Abstracts	Provides specific information and details if the Call for Abstracts is for paper or podium presentation or poster presentation. Sometimes, the Call for Podium or Paper presentations may be before the Call for Poster presentations.	Call for Abstracts: Podium and Poster Presentation
Conference Theme	The conference theme helps you determine if your scholarly work is a good fit with the conference theme. Typically, the conference themes are broad and inclusive, taking many scholarly activities into account.	*International Conference Theme: Global Healthcare Innovations: Bridging the Chasm*
Podium/ Poster Abstract Categories	The Podium/Poster Abstract Categories usually provide a range of areas for nurse scholars to share scholarly works from a variety of perspectives.	**Session 1: Best Practice Innovations: Translating Evidence in Clinical Nursing** Research studies, evidence-based projects, quality improvement projects related to clinical practice; patient safety; nursing and medical management of care in various health conditions including, but not limited to, neurological, cardiopulmonary, endocrinology, renal, genitourinary, immunology, emergencies, critical care, geriatrics, maternity and child health, psychiatry, and pediatrics.

(continued)

TABLE 9.2 Key Components for a "Call for Abstracts" *(continued)*

Key Component	Description	Example
		Session 2: Nursing Leaders Worldwide: The Future of Innovations Professional regulatory licensure requirements in the United States and the Philippines, adaptation to clinical practice settings; workforce placement of the Filipino nurses educated in the United States or Philippines; healthcare workforce, innovative leadership strategies to manage the healthcare challenges; taking the lead in resolving healthcare issues.
Guidelines for Abstract Submission	This section contains specific guidance and direction on the length of the abstract. The length is usually described, allowing a certain number of words. The font is also specified as well as contents, where to submit, how to submit, and due date.	Guidelines for Abstract Submission 1. All abstracts must be submitted to PNAAInternational@gmail.com. Please download and use the form Call for Poster/Podium Abstract Application. 2. The components of the abstract are divided into sections to help authors ensure that they have included all the required information based on the scoring criteria. Authors are encouraged to write the abstract in a word processing file (e.g., Microsoft Word). 3. The final abstract (body of abstract) must be no more than 300 words (excluding the title and authors' names). Check the word count of your abstract (excluding the title and authors' names) in a word processing program prior to sending. 4. The abstract submission will not be reviewed unless all required fields are completed (see application form below).

(continued)

TABLE 9.2 Key Components for a "Call for Abstracts" (*continued*)

Key Component	Description	Example
		5. To ensure consistent, high-quality content, all abstracts must be organized into the required format based on the abstract category.
		6. The abstract title should clearly indicate the nature of the subject. Acronyms should not be used in the title and should be written out on first mention. A quantifiable objective must be submitted and the body of the abstract should be in paragraph form, using complete sentences and avoiding special characters. Abstracts should have all funding sources written out completely if applicable.
		7. If the work is in progress, include all planned methods, projected sample size, analyses, and timeline.
		8. For abstracts with more than one author, the presenting author will be considered the contact person.
		9. Abstracts MUST be submitted on or before **April 15, 20XX.**
Abstract Headings	**Clinical/Evidence-Based Practice** • Objective • Significance and Background • Purpose • Interventions • Evaluation • Discussion	Provide guidance for specific criteria/subheadings to include in the abstract submission. The specific guidance will vary depending on the abstract heading. For example, a research abstract will differ from a clinical/evidence-based practice intervention.

Source: Adapted from Call for Abstracts. Retrieved from http://mypnaa.org/News/11th–International–Nursing–Conference–2018–Call-For-Abstract

The "call for abstracts" includes information about acceptance, notification, and if there is any delay in the notification other than what was stated earlier. Often a liaison person or member of the conference committee sends an email to those who have submitted an abstract with an updated date for notification. The successful acceptance of an abstract depends on adherence to the guidelines published by the conference sponsors.

It is important to begin working on the oral paper or poster presentation upon notification of acceptance. Do not wait until the last minute to begin this important process. Due to continuing education approvals, the conference committee will ask for submission of the presentation several weeks prior to the conference to upload into their program by a specific deadline. Missing the specified deadline may result in the inability to present at the conference.

The conference guidelines provide exact details on what to submit and how to submit the actual oral paper or poster presentation. For example, when presenting an oral paper, typically the presenter will be given a 15-minute presentation time period with 5 minutes for questions and answers. This is usually given in the form of a PowerPoint presentation and a handout for the audience. Many conferences are now paperless, and the handouts are available online prior to the conference as well as for a designated period of time following the conference.

Successful acceptance of an oral presentation or having a paper accepted for publication in a professional, peer-reviewed, scholarly journal is an honor. These are excellent strategies to disseminate one's scholarship. The key point is to learn how to properly submit an abstract in order to have the best chance of acceptance. For example, there may be hundreds of submissions that one is competing against but the more practice and experience one has in submitting one's scholarship, the more confident and competent one becomes.

PREPARATION OF A MANUSCRIPT

When submitting a manuscript as a result of one's presentation, it is essential to carefully read the editor's guidelines for submission. The first step includes downloading and carefully reading the editor's guidelines. The second step is to allow time to prepare the information well in advance of the submission due date. The final step is to adhere to submission criteria and provide all documents necessary for publication.

It is wise to do a query of the journals that are being considered in order to know if there has been a recent publication with a similar topic. Another strategy is to query a journal editor regarding his or her interest in a scholarly presentation or topic of interest. Typically, the strategy today is to send a query email to the editor. The query email to the editor should be clearly focused on the topic, excluding any extraneous verbiage. A *query letter* means that one is inquiring whether or not the editor is interested in the topic for publication (Saver, 2014, p. 49). Table 9.3 provides content as to how to write an effective query letter and rationale to do so.

It is important to complete due diligence on the timeliness and relevance of professional, peer-reviewed, scholarly work that a journal may be interested in reviewing. Review of the editorial guidelines in detail and becoming familiar with the required criteria prior to submitting an idea for review provides an opportunity to become knowledgeable about the focus of the journal. One strategy is to print the journal criteria for a manuscript submission and note all due dates.

TABLE 9.3 Components of a Query Letter to a Journal Editor

Criteria for Writing an Effective Query Email	Rationale
Review 2 to 3 years of topics and Tables of Contents for the journal you are targeting	Be certain you are not writing about a topic that has recently been published in the journal
Review the journal's focus and mission	Be certain your publication/topic is consistent with and congruent with the journal's focus and mission
Send the email query to the correct person	Be sure you carefully review the journal guidelines and follow them explicitly Take your time and get the information correct before submitting
Include correct spelling of the name and credentials of the person you are querying	You want to be correct in properly addressing the journal representative such as the editor-in-chief or associate editor-in-chief
Indicate the abstract of the article	This provides a clear, compelling, and succinct overview of the article
Provide a brief but compelling overview of your educational and experiential qualifications	This helps the editor see what knowledge, skills, and competencies you have to prepare this scholarly publication as well as your credibility to write about this topic
Include a timeline for when you could submit the manuscript	It is critical and essential that authors are professional and meet their deadlines as a professional accountability and ethical principle

TABLE 9.4 Sample Author Guidelines for Peer-Reviewed Journals

Nursing Journal	Website for Author Guidelines
Philippine Nurses Association of America, Inc. (JNPARR)	http://mypnaa.org/JNPARR/Information-for-Prospective-Authors
Journal of Public Health Management & Practice	https://jphmpdirect.com/author-guidelines
Journal of Epidemiology and Community Health	https://jech.bmj.com/pages/authors
Research in Nursing & Health	https://onlinelibrary.wiley.com/page/journal/1098240x/homepage/ForAuthors.html
Nursing Research	https://journals.lww.com/nursingresearchonline/_layouts/15/1033/oaks.journals/informationforauthors.aspx
Journal of Professional Nursing	https://www.elsevier.com/journals/journal-of-professional-nursing/8755-7223/guide-for-authors
Clinical Nursing Research	https://us.sagepub.com/en-us/nam/journal-author-gateway

The second step would be to write notes for clarification or questions to ask the editor if there are any uncertainties. Journal editors are interested in new ideas and are happy to offer guidance and support for new and innovative manuscripts. Table 9.4 provides a sample of author guidelines.

PEER-REVIEW PROCESS FOR PUBLICATION

Once the journal receives a new article, it will be sent to selected members of their editorial board for review. Typically, the journal has two educationally and experientially qualified peer reviewers for the article. The selected members of the editorial board read and score the submission using a standard rubric. Peer reviewers try to offer comments along with a score on a standard rubric. The outcome of the editorial review is to determine if the submission is publishable as is, or if the submission requires minor revision and resubmission, or if the submission requires major revision and resubmission.

Each peer-reviewed journal has a specified time frame that is used to hold peer reviewers accountable to meet deadlines so that manuscripts can be returned to the author(s) in a timely manner. For example, when a peer reviewer is asked to review a manuscript, he or she is

BOX 9.1 Sample Communication to a Peer Reviewer

On 27/Jul/20XX, you kindly agreed to review the above-referenced manuscript. This is a friendly reminder that your review of this manuscript is due by 10/Aug/20XX.

provided a deadline for the manuscript review. The typical deadline for a manuscript review is 2 to 3 weeks or 15 business days. A sample communication to a peer reviewer and response to a manuscript has been exemplified in Box 9.1.

Once the peer review is complete, the peer reviewers typically receive an email regarding the decision by the journal editor to publish or not. There are several manuscript decisions that may be used when a manuscript has been reviewed. Table 9.5 provides examples of decisions that may be used from a peer-reviewed journal.

The true challenge to receiving peer-review feedback is accepting and receiving the feedback and using that feedback to help modify or revise the submission toward acceptance. Journal editors and peer reviewers try to offer positive, supportive guidance to the author(s) (Terharr & Sylvan, 2016). The feedback is not intended to be demeaning or to ridicule an aspiring author. Rather, the peer-review process is intended to offer positive guidance and support that encourages future submissions.

Often, peer-reviewed feedback on a manuscript provides a brief summary of the manuscript as submitted, summarizing the peer reviewer's perception of the manuscript in his or her words. The criteria and feedback for a peer reviewer's perception of the manuscript may include the following content:

- Main impressions of the manuscript: Is the manuscript timely and relevant?
- Is the manuscript adding to the knowledge base and science?
- Is the article timely, relevant, and contemporary?
- Does the abstract accurately reflect the article content in a clear and succinct manner?
- Is there a strong statement of purpose at the end of the first or second paragraph telling readers what to expect as they read the manuscript?
- What is the main theme or focus of the manuscript?
- Does the title accurately reflect the content of the manuscript?
- Does all information in the manuscript support the main theme or focus of the manuscript?

TABLE 9.5 Examples of Manuscript Decisions From a Peer-Reviewed Journal

Manuscript Decisions	Implications of the Decision
1. Accept as submitted	No changes are needed. The manuscript is accepted for publication as is.
2. Accept with minor revision	The peer review means peer reviewers agree on the manuscript as a good fit with their journal. The changes needed typically are described in the form of comments in the original manuscript or in a comment section of the journal's standard rubric so that the author(s) of the article know specifically what changes need to be made for resubmission and successful chance of publication. There is typically a timeline specified in which the minor revisions need to be made and a resubmission deadline. It is critical to meet the resubmission deadline. The article will typically be re-reviewed by peer reviewers. The re-review may occur by the peer reviewers who initially reviewed the article or the resubmission may be reviewed by new peer reviewers. The re-review process typically takes the same amount of time as the initial peer review of the article.
3. Accept with major revision	The peer review means peer reviewers found major issues with the manuscript as submitted. Even with major revision, the manuscript has potential but will require a substantive amount of work and revision. Just like a manuscript that is accepted with minor revision, the peer reviewers and journal editor provide detailed information on what needs to be changed or updated to have a publishable manuscript. There is typically a timeline specified in which the minor revisions need to be made and a resubmission deadline. It is critical to meet the resubmission deadline. The article will typically be re-reviewed by peer reviewers. The re-review may occur by the peer reviewers who initially reviewed the article or the resubmission may be reviewed by new peer reviewers. The re-review process typically takes the same amount of time as the initial peer review of the article.
4. Reject	The journal editor reviews the peer reviews. The journal editor examines the manuscript to be sure the manuscript meets the journal editorial/author guidelines. For example, if the manuscript is too long and exceeds the journal specifications for the length of the manuscript, the manuscript will not be accepted. If the manuscript title is to be a certain number of characters or words, the manuscript must adhere to those guidelines. The peer review focuses on editorial/journal guidelines as well as peer review to see the "goodness of fit" and degree to which the peer reviewers determine the manuscript meets editorial guidelines for the journal.

- Are all references current (within the past 5 years) and relevant to support the main theme or focus of the manuscript?
- Are the sections of the manuscript clearly labeled in proper format as specified by the editorial/author guidelines? For example, if the guidelines indicate American Psychological Association (APA) format, there should be level 1 and/or level 2 subheadings in proper APA format.
- Is the manuscript the proper length according to editorial/ author guidelines?
- Is the manuscript in the proper font and size according to editorial/author guidelines?

It is unlikely that a manuscript submission will be accepted without some type of revision on the first submission. One of the challenges with a manuscript that requires major or minor revisions is that there is not a guarantee that the manuscript will meet publication requirements even after major or minor revision(s) and resubmission. Another major challenge with feedback indicating minor revision, major revision, or rejection is that authors may "give up." It is not uncommon to have feelings of despair and frustration after working diligently on a manuscript and getting feedback that the manuscript needs minor revision or major revision, or is rejected. The key is not to despair, not to feel rejection, not to take the feedback personally, and not to give up. The key to becoming a successful author and scholar is to embrace the feedback provided to improve one's work and to keep on working diligently in order to turn the submission into a premier publishable manuscript.

WHERE TO SUBMIT FOR PUBLICATION

The purpose of submitting DNP scholarship for publication is to translate and disseminate evidence-based research into clinical practice. Translation of research into practice, dissemination, and integration of new knowledge are key activities of DNP graduates (American Association of Colleges of Nursing [AACN], 2006). DNP graduates are expected to engage in advanced nursing practice as well as provide leadership for evidence-based practice (AACN, 2006, p. 11). DNP students need to understand that it is not acceptable to submit their final DNP project paper to a professional, peer-reviewed journal for publication in its present format. The final DNP project paper is not the same as a publication-ready article.

DNP students should search for journals that publish quality improvement articles and that have readers who would be interested in findings from DNP projects. DNP students need to follow the author guidelines and format their papers accordingly, prior to submitting to the journal. Adhering strictly to the editorial guidelines will provide greater success for acceptance of the manuscript. Additionally, it is best not to submit the same manuscript to multiple journals or multiple conferences at the same time. Submitting the same manuscript to a variety of journals results in duplicity and often negatively impacts on one's ability to publish. Thus, it is best to receive feedback from each journal one at a time. Be selective about where to submit your scholarly work and pay attention to every detail to enhance the chance for success rather than submit your work to multiple venues at the same time.

DNP students wishing to publish in a professional, peer-reviewed scholarly journal should compute the "impact factor" related to the topic of interest. This is important because it allows the DNP student to understand how his or her manuscript topic would be accepted by others. The "impact factor" of a journal article provides a measure of the frequency that the journal article has been cited in other peer-reviewed scholarly articles in a specific year. Most librarians are able to help you conduct a search to determine a specific journal and its impact factor. The impact factor is a very important concept for authors deciding where to publish their scholarly works.

The impact factor is based on the calculation of how many times the article has been cited in the previous 2 years. The impact factor is important for a variety of reasons. For example, for researchers or faculty members seeking promotion and/or tenure, this is very important when their work is reviewed by peers. The higher the number for the impact factor, the more rigorous and prestigious the journal. For example, the scientific journal *Nature* has an impact factor of 40, making it a very prestigious journal to have an accepted publication.

Computation of "impact factor" for an article published in 2016 would be computed by a numerator of the number of times articles were cited in 2014–2015 in indexed journals during 2016 divided by the denominator consisting of the number of citable publications published in 2014–2015 (Saver, 2014, p. 47). For example, an impact factor of 1.0 means that articles published from 2014–2015 were cited one time. *The Journal for Nurse Practitioners* has an impact factor of 0.487 and the *International Journal of Nursing Studies* has an impact factor of 3.656. The impact factor should always be a consideration when deciding where to publish one's scholarly project.

Finally, it is important to strictly adhere to the author guidelines that are provided by the journal editors. Journal editors do not want to receive a manuscript that does not meet their editorial and author guidelines. For example, if the guidelines require the manuscript to be no more than 4,500 words and the manuscript is 4,800, the manuscript may be rejected. Many online submission software products used for submission of scholarly work(s) will not allow submission if specific editorial or author guidelines are not met. For example, if the title can only be 15 words and the title is 17 words, the software will indicate an error and you must adjust the number of words in the title before successfully submitting. Thus, it is important to review the focus of the journal of interest, editorial guidelines, readership, and topics so that one's scholarly work is more likely to be accepted for a publication.

WHERE *NOT* TO SUBMIT FOR SCHOLARLY PUBLICATION

Currently, there are more and more predatory or journal conferences being advertised and available. Often, these journals or conferences appear as legitimate peer-reviewed, scholarly places to publish or to present one's scholarship (McCann & Polacsek, 2018). A predatory journal/conference is one that violates acceptable standards and ethical principles for scholarly publications or presentations (Butler, 2013). In 2014, the International Academy of Nursing Editors (INANE) became concerned about the issue of open-access journals and predatory journals that appeared to be eroding scholarly standards. The old saying "If it's too good to be true, it usually is" pertains to some open-access journals and predatory journals. For example, many open-access and predatory journals charge a fee of thousands of dollars to publish. Box 9.2 provides a list of characteristics that are often found with predatory journals or conferences that seek manuscripts or presentations from professionals.

Open-access journals are wonderful; however, the open-access journal may fall short and erode the evidence-based science and

BOX 9.2 Characteristics of Predatory Journals/Conferences

- Charges a fee that can be several thousand dollars for the privilege to publish one's scholarly work
- Features speakers/writers who are recruited by email, not vetted by leading scholars and academics
- Typically, anyone who pays gets a spot on the podium, which used to embellish or pad one's résumé
- Online/open-access journals that print anything for a fee
- Email solicitations regarding a publishing opportunity that is "too good to be true"

nursing scholarship. The following link provides excellent information on open-access publishing (OAP), predatory publishing, author's rights, and open educational resources (OERs): qcc.libguides.com/open/predatorypublishing

WHEN TO SUBMIT FOR PUBLICATION

It is important to submit scholarly work that is timely, relevant, and contemporary. Waiting to publish one's DNP scholarly project results in outdated or untimely information that may no longer be relevant in the clinical or practice setting. The idea behind scholarly presentations or submissions is to get the scholarship into practice as soon as possible. Delaying or waiting to publish or present one's scholarly work means the references will be quickly outdated and the review of the literature will need to be updated. The DNP student may have multiple scholarly presentations or publications from one DNP project. For example, the DNP student may want to submit one paper focusing on a systematic review of the literature conducted for the DNP project and a second paper or presentation on the best evidence for an intervention resulting from the project. The idea is that the publication or presentation consists of sharing scholarly work that is timely, relevant, and contemporary to help improve patient care, inform executive leaders, and to provide content consistent with patient safety and quality patient care.

HOW TO SUBMIT FOR PUBLICATION

As previously discussed, it is important to review the editor or author guidelines. There is information on the journal's website about the type of manuscripts that are accepted as well as the major focus of the journal. Submission guidelines are typically well described on the website or in the journal for specific submission guidelines. Following the specific author guidelines prior to submitting one's work will assist in more positive outcomes.

EDITORIAL RESPONSES TO SUBMITTED PUBLICATIONS

One of the most exciting components to the submission of a professional manuscript is to wait for the results of a submitted manuscript. Regardless of the type of scholarship submitted, the submission guidelines will provide a notification date. Often, the editor will provide feedback to the author within a given time period. Once one is notified about the manuscript submission, one will have time to respond to the editor's comments. If one receives notification as to acceptance of a manuscript with minor editorial changes, one will have time to respond and resubmit the manuscript. If one has major changes, additional materials may have to be sent along with rewrites that have been required by the editor. If the manuscript was not accepted, the editor will provide feedback as to how to revise or rework your manuscript. Rejection of a manuscript does not mean that it cannot be resubmitted to another journal; often, it means that the topic or how it was written did not meet the criteria for their particular journal. Exhibit 9.2 provides an example of a manuscript that was rejected from a peer-reviewed journal.

EXHIBIT 9.2 Example of a Manuscript That Was Rejected From a Peer-Reviewed Journal

Sample Feedback Received From a Manuscript Submission That Was Rejected
Article Summary

The focus of this article is on XXX XXX. The article highlights XXX XXX. The article includes XXX XXX.

My main impressions of the article are that it is a novel topic with an interesting focus, addressing several issues focusing on XXX XXX.
The article could be more compelling and add to the knowledge base with strengthening the abstract to more accurately reflect the content of the article. I do not think the abstract accurately reflects the article content in a clear and succinct manner. The abstract is not complete and "stand-alone" as submitted.
The article appears to conform to the journal-specific instructions and guide for authors. The abstract needs to have a strong statement of what the article is about.
The introductory paragraph tends to be a bit too general, lacking needed details and specificity. For example, ...

- The title does not accurately reflect the content. For example, the current title is XXX XXX, while the article appears to be more about XXX XXX.

(continued)

- The portion of the article about XXX is not really the main theme or main idea for this article. The main theme to me is XXX XXX There are multiple main ideas in the article as submitted.
- The discussion/conclusion and references appear to be a bit dated, and references should be within the past 5 years for the most part.
- Facts and presentation of concepts in the article need to be organized with level 1 subheadings according to the concepts.

The conclusions are not well supported by the data in the article as presented.

Regardless of the type of notification one receives from the editor, what is important is that the development of one's own scholarship requires hard work and the ability to promote one's work so that others can cite the work and be accepted as a peer. The importance of feedback both orally and written provides the foundation for the development of a scholar. Professional growth as a DNP scholar takes experience, time, and the ability to become a lifelong learner. It is important to continue to provide the evidence-based research needed to advance the profession of nursing through quality and innovative clinical innovations.

SUMMARY

The purpose to disseminate the results of the DNP project and report the results to the stakeholders, academic communities of interest, and healthcare professionals remains the most important attribute when completing the DNP project. Regardless of the results of the DNP project it is important to share these results since others may have identified comparable problems or may want to replicate the project. The focus of this chapter was to understand the relevance and importance of committing to a scholarly trajectory upon completion of the DNP program. Specifically, this chapter identified and described strategies and best practices to disseminate DNP scholarship in a variety of ways. For example, there is emphasis on how to present material via oral or written presentations at local, regional, and national programs. A focus on the importance of formatting, adhering to presentation guidelines, and following author guidelines was presented. Additionally, content has been reviewed and described specifically about peer-review processes, manuscript or presentation of projects, authorship, and contributions by the committee members. The application of how a DNP student is able to present and disseminate his or her DNP project findings was discussed.

APPLICATION EXERCISES: DEVELOPMENT OF A MEANINGFUL POSTER PRESENTATION

Introduction

Poster presentations are visual presentations of a scientific report, an evidence-based quality assurance project, or a case report that is used to determine a new method for clinical interventions. Most professional meetings provide time for poster presentations. When a poster is accepted at a professional conference, it undergoes a peer-review process to determine if it meets the guidelines and standards determined by the review committee.

There are a few basic principles to keep in mind as to how to develop a professional poster presentation. Designing the poster includes a visual presentation that allows the reader to easily review the content without difficulty. For example, it is best to follow the conference guidelines when preparing a poster presentation. The following tips can assist in the development of a poster:

- Leave adequate white space to promote legibility.
- Use plain, descriptive language allowing the data to be read from left to right.
- Use visual images when available such as photos, illustrations, or graphs since people retain images longer than words.
- Make it readable by using letters or fonts that are clear enough so that the participants can view it without difficulty.
- Use peer review by asking colleagues to review your draft for clarity or possible errors.

A poster presentation should present the essential content about the topic; thus, it is best to organize one's thoughts and develop the content that is consistent with the most important aspects of the project. Using these guidelines will assist in the development of a well-written poster.

As a new DNP graduate, it is important to begin to develop recognition of one's scholarly work or clinical expertise. One way to become skilled at becoming a DNP scholar is to apply for poster presentations at local, regional, and national professional meetings. Attendance at these professional meetings will provide networking opportunities and assist in the further development of one's clinical area of expertise.

Case Presentation

Susie was asked to represent her hospital at a regional research meeting and complete a poster presentation related to evidence-based practice and use of research in the clinical setting. Susie is in her second semester of her DNP program and has not completed her coursework. However, she has been working at a local hospital as a clinical supervisor at a busy ambulatory care setting. Susie has done numerous clinical teaching sessions at the hospital; however, she has not presented at a professional meeting. Since she is new at this process, she feels insecure and apprehensive. Because her director of nursing is impressed with her clinical competencies, she wants to be sure that she represents her hospital organization well and be able to teach her staff how to complete a poster presentation in the future. Susie has chosen to present a topic related to the use of evidence-based practice approaches associated with patient education in an ambulatory care setting.

Application Exercise Questions

1. What are the first steps that Susie should consider to prepare a professional poster at a regional meeting?
2. Should Susie consider having other staff nurses involved in the development of the poster presentation?
3. What is the purpose of poster presentations at professional meetings?
4. Where will Susie locate information about completing a poster presentation?
5. What are the key components of a poster presentation?
6. How will Susie overcome her anxiety or challenges related to presenting at a professional meeting?
7. Examine how participating in a poster presentation may be useful to one's professional growth as a scholar?
8. How are poster presentations evaluated? Discuss possible criteria.

REFERENCES

American Association of Colleges of Nursing. (2006). *The essentials of doctoral education for advanced nursing practice.* Retrieved from http://www .aacnnursing.org/Portals/42/Publications/DNPEssentials.pdf
Boyer, E. (1997). *Scholarship reconsidered: Priorities of the professoriate.* San Francisco, CA: Jossey-Bass.

Brown, M. A., & Crabtree, K. (2013). The development of practice scholarship in DNP programs: A paradigm shift. *Journal of Professional Nursing, 29,* 330–337. doi:10.1016/j.profnurs.2013.08.003

Butler, D. (2013). Investigating journals: The dark side of publishing. *Nature, 495,* 434–435.

McCann, T. V., & Polacsek, M. (2018). False gold: Safely navigating open access publishing to avoid predatory publishers and journals. *Journal of Advanced Nursing, 74*(4), 809–817. doi:10.1111/jan.13483

Saver, C. (2014). *Anatomy of writing for publication for nurses* (2nd ed., p. 49). Indianapolis, IN: Sigma Theta Tau International.

Terhaar, M., & Sylvia, M. (2016). Scholarly work products of the doctor of nursing practice: One approach to evaluating scholarship, rigor, impact and quality. *Journal of Clinical Nursing, 25,* 163–174. doi:10.1111/jocn.13113.

10 AFTER THE PROJECT: INCORPORATING KNOWLEDGE INTO A SUCCESSFUL CAREER

DENISE M. KORNIEWICZ

INTRODUCTION

Once the DNP project has been successfully completed, it is not unusual to put the written project on a shelf and not look at it again because the goal of the DNP program was to complete a successful project and obtain the clinical doctoral degree. However, the findings associated with the project allow others to learn and improve their clinical practice. Thus, it is important to focus on how to continue one's clinical scholarship as one transitions from a novice to an expert APRN. The transition from an APRN student to an expert APRN can be conceptualized within Pat Benner's "novice to expert" nursing model (Benner, 1984); see Table 10.1 (Korniewicz, 2015).

The evolution from the role of a student APRN to an expert APRN may be described in much the same way that Benner (1984) described novice nurses as they entered into clinical practice. Often, the new APRNs when entering into a new clinical site may display behaviors such as lack of confidence, marginal clinical performance skills, and the inability to adhere to specific appointment times. These characteristics are consistent with the professional development of a novice APRN and are expected as one becomes more knowledgeable and proficient within their new role. It may take months to years before a new APRN graduate becomes an expert APRN. Attributes such as confidence, clinical competence, accuracy in managing a patient caseload, and the ability to

TABLE 10.1 Application of Pat Benner's Model for Advanced Practice Practitioners (1984)

Stages of Development	Definition	Examples of an APRN's Stages of Development	Expected Outcomes Based on Stages and Clinical Expertise
Novice	The novice or beginner has no experience with what he or she is expected to perform. Lacks confidence and practice is more prolonged because of learning new role.	• New graduate from an advanced practice program. • Takes more time in the assessment of the patient.	• Reads literature consistent with safe clinical practice.
Advanced beginner	Demonstrates marginally acceptable performance because of prior clinical preceptorship during the clinical program. May have delayed time periods while providing care.	• Demonstrates acceptable beginning level skills associated with the assessment and management of patients. • Level of management is beginning to develop.	• Involved in peer review of clinical patient load. • Discusses alternate treatment methods.
Competent	Demonstrates efficiency, coordination of caseload, and has confidence in actions. Establishes a skill level consistent with the efficiency of an APRN who has been practicing 2–3 years. Patients are seen in an efficient and suitable time frame.	• Demonstrates confidence and safety by knowing when to discuss a patient's clinical problem with peers. • Carries an appropriate number of clinic patients and provides timely and proficient care.	• Provides leadership to others through clinical rounds and participates in interdisciplinary peer review. • Participates in developing clinical scholarship through development of clinical protocols or case reports.

(continued)

TABLE 10.1 Application of Pat Benner's Model for Advanced Practice Practitioners (1984) *(continued)*

Stages of Development	Definition	Examples of an APRN's Stages of Development	Expected Outcomes Based on Stages and Clinical Expertise
Proficiency	Demonstrates an understanding of patient problems as a whole versus segments. The proficient advanced practice practitioner learns from experience, readily suggests practice changes or interventions, and makes clear decisions based on the standards related to safe clinical practice.	• Develops new practice guidelines consistent with specialty area. • Provides leadership to other healthcare providers in the management of patient care.	• Participates in the publication of clinical manuscripts relevant to his or her specialty. • Leads others in the development of new healthcare delivery models. • Presentation at interdisciplinary conferences.
Expert	Demonstrates accuracy in the assessment of patient problems and is skillful at diagnosis and management. Highly skilled analytic ability is demonstrated and proficient, timely performance is demonstrated via peer review.	• Accurate diagnosis, treatment, and management of patients. • Works independently and consults only when necessary. • Teaches or precepts others.	• Participates in all peer-review processes. • Independently publishes or suggests revision of clinical protocols.

Source: From Korniewicz, D. (2015). *Nursing leadership and management: The advanced practice role.* Lancaster, PA: DEStech Publications, Inc.

provide proficient evidence-based patient care provide the foundation for expert clinical practice and can assist in the transition period from novice to expert APRN practice.

Although it may be difficult to adjust to the APRN role, it is just as important to determine how one views one's own contributions to the nursing profession. The importance of improving clinical care and developing clinical practice models that can be used to change or improve the overall quality of patient care is an important aspect of one's own clinical scholarship. This chapter provides the steps needed to understand how to become a clinical scholar, how to grow as a clinical scholar, how to become a lifelong learner, how to develop one's own goals as a clinical scholar, and how to contribute as a clinical scholar. Finally, this step-by-step approach to clinical scholarship will assist in the development as an expert APRN and provide the foundation for lifelong learning.

DEFINING CLINICAL SCHOLARSHIP

The investigation into defining clinical scholarship was initially undertaken by the Clinical Scholarship Task Force, Sigma Theta Tau International (1999). This task force was able to differentiate between research and clinical practice by providing a set of characteristics associated with clinical inquiry. The characteristics included a set of clinical quality indicators that measured the effectiveness of patient outcomes, accountability for clinical work, and the ability to solve clinical problems and to develop new products or services that were patient centered or population based. Additionally, the need to function collaboratively within interdisciplinary teams (Sigma Theta Tau, 1999) was considered an essential component of clinical scholarship.

The definition of clinical scholarship was further expanded in 1999 by the American Association of Colleges of Nursing (AACN) as:

> . . . those activities that systematically advance the teaching, research, and practice of nursing through rigorous inquiry that (1) is significant to the profession, (2) is creative, (3) can be documented, (4) can be replicated or elaborated, and can be peer-reviewed through various methods. (AACN, 1999)

Today, the AACN has provided clear guidelines associated with clinical scholarship to include patient outcome management, quality improvement, and evidence-based clinical practice projects that translate evidence into practice or policy to improve patient care. Furthermore, the National Organization of APRN Faculties (NONPF, 2016) has defined the characteristics of APRN clinical scholars as lifelong learners who use evidence-based practice skills to translate the current best clinical evidence into practice guidelines that improve patient care and provide healthcare outcomes that transform systems of care. Thus, APRNs have been educated to translate research into practice and direct evaluation processes to determine if the research has had any impact on the development, implementation, or evaluation of new or improved models of care.

As a novice APRN, it is difficult to define one's own definition of a clinical scholar. Often, beginning APRNs do not view themselves as clinical scholars; however, through self-reflection one can determine the attributes associated with one's own clinical scholarship. Examples may include one's extensive experiences in clinical practice such as skilled observation, extensive treatment knowledge, ability to critically think and analyze a clinical situation, and determine the best practice associated with a clinical problem. Developing one's ability to integrate intellectual curiosity and scholarly inquiry provides the basis to determine the next steps in providing the clinical management and leadership necessary to contribute as an APRN and clinical scholar.

Perhaps, it is best to describe the novice clinical scholar as one who identifies the best practices associated with the health options available for a set population; for example, acute versus chronic illness or pediatric versus geriatric care providers. The building blocks associated with identifying and developing one's area of clinical scholarship may include: (a) development of annual goals related to the population served; (b) identification of the clinical area of interest for the population or community served; (c) critical analysis of the health and wellness options available for the clinical area of interest or population; (d) development of a matrix associated with clinical questions that remain unanswered about the population served; and (e) examination of future questions related to the clinical area of interest or population. The key point for the novice APRN to consider is to always ask "why" or "how" in order to continue to learn from the patient or other healthcare providers about their health population of interest. Once novice APRNs begin to view or review their patient population as a way to develop innovative or creative avenues for clinical care, then it becomes easier to develop their own road map of clinical scholarship (Figure 10.1).

CULTIVATING ONE'S OWN CLINICAL SCHOLARSHIP

As the novice APRN begins to develop and grow as an expert APRN, questions may arise about one's own clinical scholarship. Examples may include: (a) Where do I fit as a clinical scholar? (b) To date, what

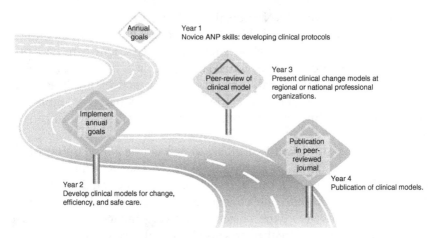

FIGURE 10.1 Road map for clinical scholarship.

ANP, advanced nurse practitioner.

are my best clinical accomplishments? (c) Can I suggest an innovative change in our clinical practice routines? (d) Will I be able to handle peer review of my ideas? (e) Will I be able to contribute through publication? Perhaps one way to contemplate how to answer these questions would be to review one's own knowledge, skills, and attitudes associated with a clinical issue; for example, understanding that research primarily informs clinical practice of theoretical issues while clinical practice generates questions about the clinical problem. Often the clinical question is the foundational building block for further clinical inquiry. Exploring the clinical question by reviewing the evidence in the literature, critically appraising the validity of the research, and applying findings to make a clinical decision are all components of evidence-based practice. Using an evidence-based practice approach to investigate a clinical problem will provide a process that will assist in the further development of a clinical scholar.

In order to define one's own clinical scholarship, it is important to understand the competencies needed to make evidence-based clinical decisions. Clinical decisions may range from fast, intuitive decisions to well thought out or evidence based. The competencies needed to differentiate between simple and complex clinical decision-making practices include core values and skills that integrate problem-solving abilities with effective and core values associated with safe patient care. These competencies may include (a) pattern recognition, (b) critical thinking, (c) communication, (d) use of evidence-based approaches, (e) teamwork, (f) ability to share results, and (g) use of reflection (Chapa, Hartung, Mayberry, & Pintz, 2013). Clinical decision-making includes the application of competencies that promote expert problem-solving abilities and tend to support one's ability to become a clinical scholar. Application of each of these competencies may include a list of actions or performance measures that can be targeted as monthly or annual goals (Table 10.2).

Finally, it is the application of evidence-based practice models that distinguishes the APRN as a clinical scholar versus an APRN who does not base his or her practice on a foundational model of scientific inquiry. The development of clinical scholarship is dependent on using scientific databases to define the clinical question and assist the APRN to further develop the patient outcomes associated with the clinical problem. At this point, it is the translation of the clinical question into everyday clinical practice that is the most important aspect to be considered. The clinical scholar needs to apply new knowledge or demonstrate more

TABLE 10.2 Clinical Decision-Making Competencies, Definitions, and Actions for Clinical Scholars

Competency	Definition	Action or Performance Measures for Clinical Scholars
Pattern recognition	Learning from clinical experiences	Ability to define best practices in the clinical setting for the defined population
Communication	Patient-centered approaches, active listening	Provides change to clinical practice through development of new ways to care for the patient population
Evidence-based approaches	Uses most current clinical guidelines	Implements changes that reflect national standards for the patient population
Teamwork	Gathers advice and evidence from other healthcare teams	Obtains input from peers to develop new clinical models and obtains critical feedback to make changes
Ability to share results	Reflects on decisions to improve patient care	Evaluates peer-review changes to provide quality patient care
Use of reflection	Obtains local, regional, and national feedback to improve patient care	Presents patient outcome data or changes to other healthcare providers via written or oral presentations to implement patient care changes

effective or efficient knowledge about a clinical problem. Application of the science and integration of the clinical effectiveness or results will provide the best solution to the clinical problem. The overall goal of the clinical scholar will be to continually learn and disseminate new or more proficient clinical care by providing more effective patient care outcomes. One of the many attributes of a clinical scholar is the ability to become a lifelong learner and be open to changes within the clinical practice setting.

LIFELONG LEARNING AND CLINICAL SCHOLARSHIP

It is clear within the NONPF guidelines that the APRN is characterized as an individual who promotes the characteristics of lifelong learning. In order to understand how to implement these characteristics, one has to understand the overall principles associated with lifelong learning. Several authors (Kellenberg, Schmidt, & Werner, 2017; Patra, 2010) have conceptualized the characteristics of lifelong learners as individuals who have the following qualities: (a) thirst for knowledge; (b) goal directed; (c) passion for learning; (d) inquisitive; and (e) curious. Attributes that have been used to describe lifelong learners include motivation and the interest in education, competence to apply knowledge successfully, self-determination, self-regulation, and reflective learning experiences (Homayounzadeh, 2016). Therefore, APRNs who are lifelong learners consistently seek out answers to clinical questions and are leaders who are involved in critiquing and integrating evidence-based approaches into everyday clinical practice.

Lifelong learning is especially needed by healthcare professionals because their work involves human life. To provide high-quality nursing care that protects and preserves life, nurses and other healthcare professionals should keep abreast of scientific developments (Hojat, Veloski, & Gonnela, 2009; Longworth, 2003). Examples as to how APRNs as lifelong learners can be engaged in improving clinical practice would include: (a) validating individual practice and competence; (b) engaging others in new knowledge and skill acquisition; (c) participating in the identification of clinical performance gaps; (d) expanding or/and improving patient-centered clinical outcomes; (e) incorporating knowledge, skills, performance, competence, and judgment when working with patient populations; and (f) developing ways to prevent burnout by using preventive methods related to self-satisfaction. APRNs become clinical scholars as a result of their continued interest to provide quality patient care and their ability to quickly integrate new knowledge into clinical practice.

Successful lifelong-learning APRNs who become clinical scholars view knowledge and the creation of new knowledge as important to the development of quality patient care. Lüftenegger et al. (2012) found that lifelong learners have the ability to autonomously regulate their own learning and effectively manage their acquired knowledge through self-determination, self-regulation, and autonomy. Therefore, as one develops his or her clinical scholarship, it would be important to be involved in reading up-to-date treatment options, become involved in interdisciplinary healthcare discussion groups related to practice guidelines, and suggest new ways to provide evidence-based patient care.

ROAD MAP FOR CLINICAL SCHOLARSHIP

The road map for clinical scholarship includes self-reflection of one's own clinical goals and the ability to focus on the scientific attributes needed to reflect on clinical practice, and to systematically evaluate clinical practice models of care. Each step in this process requires the identification of clinical goals consistent with the growth and maturity of professional practice skills associated with APRNs. For example, realistic goals that could be developed for the clinical scholar would include annual evaluation of one's scholarly productivity. Have you identified your annual goals toward clinical scholarship? This may simply include developing new clinical protocols for your patient population or developing and presenting a new model of clinical care. Depending on one's own goals as an APRN, organizational requirements and contributions to the overall APRN profession will assist in determining one's own clinical scholarship. Perhaps, developing yearly goals or a personal road map for one's own clinical scholarship would assist in the steps from a novice to an expert clinical scholar (Figure 10.1).

One's own personal road map for a successful clinical scholarship journey may begin with the development of a new clinical model that would provide better patient care efficiencies or improve patient safety. For example, working within a specific population allows one to be more proficient and an expert while providing care. In order to identify if one is doing something unique at one's practice site, a review of local and national clinical guidelines related to treatment options would assist in obtaining the best evidence for practice.

The development of something new requires the ability to understand what has been done in the past, what is currently being done, and what could be done to make any improvements. It is important to continually question current practices in order to modify clinical care. This process provides the foundation of clinical inquiry and begins the building blocks of change or the development of new practice models. Clinical inquiry leads to the development of new clinical knowledge and promotes added experience in clinical judgment. Thus, it is through the continuous development of clinical inquiry that new or progressive clinical change occurs.

The second goal to achieve in the development of one's clinical scholarship road map is to obtain a peer review of the clinical model or changes that are of interest to one's practice site. Peer review may begin with a discussion with colleagues where one is employed and consist of issues associated with patient care. Once feedback is obtained from peers, it would be best to present ideas to your local, regional, or national professional APRN organizations to obtain additional peer review. Often, this requires submission of an abstract for written or oral presentation. However, the input from one's peers assists in the further development of an idea and often makes the clinical idea stronger because of the clinical discussions that occurred. Peer review provides a network of colleagues that can be used to further develop one's ideas or assist in the adaptation of a new clinical model.

The final goal of one's clinical road map is publication of clinical scholarship. There are three main reasons to publish as a clinical scholar: (a) to share clinical expertise with other APRNs and healthcare providers; (b) to disseminate clinical evidence-based approaches to patient care; and (c) to develop one's own knowledge and skills. Often, peer-reviewed publications can be intimidating since they require editing, rewrites, resubmission, or rejection. First-time authors often find it difficult to write for a peer-reviewed journal; however, clinical scholarship requires recognition by peers to validate new ideas. Publication provides the avenue to disseminate new ideas about your clinical scholarship. There are many references as to how to get started or how to write as a professional clinical scholar. However, what is essential and most successful is to develop a timeline and an outline of the essential content that is needed for the journal that you choose for publication. Figure 10.2 provides the steps and an example of a timeline to assist in writing for a peer-reviewed clinical journal article.

EXAMPLES OF A CLINICAL SCHOLAR

The success of a clinical scholar can be measured in a variety of ways. First and foremost, it is through the recognition of one's scholarly work by peers or other health professionals. Examples may include publications in peer-reviewed journals, presentation of innovative clinical models at annual national or international conferences, or appointment

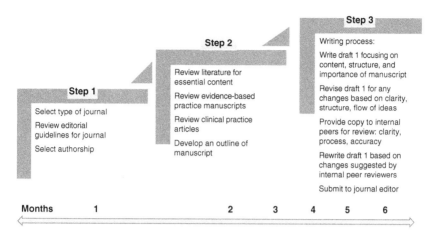

FIGURE 10.2 Steps for clinical journal publication and example of a timeline.

to national committees that develop clinical standards or guidelines. Clinical scholars have contributed to practice changes that have impacted on treatment methods for patient populations or have suggested new prevention strategies for a group of patients. Often, clinical scholars are renowned in their area of expertise and participate independently in the review of established clinical protocols, lead others in the development of new healthcare delivery models, or are proficient in mentoring others in their area of clinical expertise.

Historically, Dr. Loretta Ford (Gardenier, 2014) has been credited with beginning the APRN movement. Dr. Ford's initial clinical practice as an independent pediatric APRN is one example of a renowned clinical scholar. In 1965, she was instrumental in developing the first pediatric APRN program at the University of Colorado and was a pioneer in developing primary care services in rural health communities (Gardenier, 2014). Even today, Dr. Ford continues to be a clinical scholar through speaking engagements that address new clinical models of care and the application of technology in healthcare settings. Examples of Dr. Ford's clinical scholarship achievements can be found at the following website: www.womenofthehall.org/inductee/loretta-c-ford. The importance of Dr. Ford's work provides a clear example of how one's contributions to clinical practice can impact not only on the profession of nursing but on the lives of patients.

Perhaps one's contribution as an expert clinical scholar will not be as profound as Dr. Loretta Ford's; however, what is important is that one continually strives to develop innovative clinical pathways that lead others toward the development of new knowledge. It is the work of APRNs today who are helping to change healthcare systems because of their skills associated with quality patient care and performance measures that provide the data necessary to improve patient treatment options. Furthermore, the ability to mentor others in a clinical practice role and provide the leadership necessary to change outdated clinical models is just as important at the local level as it is at the national level. All APRNs should consider integrating the clinical nurse scholar role into their daily practice.

SUMMARY

This chapter provided the principles and attributes associated with clinical scholarship. By providing a step-by-step process in the journey toward clinical scholarship, this chapter contained the essential content required to be a successful clinical scholar. Furthermore, this chapter emphasized the need to foster lifelong learning skills and to contribute to the further development of the profession of nursing through the peer-review process of presentations and publications. Finally, a road map of annual goals was presented to guide the APRN toward a successful path for becoming a clinical scholar.

REFERENCES

American Association of Colleges of Nursing. (1999). *Statement on defining scholarship for the discipline of nursing.* Retrieved from http://www.aacnnursing.org/NewsInformation/Position-Statements-White-Papers/Defining-Scholarship-Nursing

Benner, P. (1984). *From novice to expert: Excellence and power in clinical nursing practice* (pp. 13–34). Menlo Park, CA: Addison-Wesley.

Chapa, D., Hartung, M., Mayberry, L., & Pintz, C. (2013). Using preappraised evidence sources to guide practice decisions. *Journal of the American Association of Nurse Practitioners, 25,* 234–243. doi:10.1111/j.1745-7599.2012.00787.x

Gardenier, D. (2014). 48 hours with Loretta Ford. *The Journal for Nurse Practitioners, 10*(7), 521–523. doi:10.1016/j.nurpra.2014.02.007

Hojat, M., Veloski, J. J., & Gonnela, J. S. (2009). Measurements and correlates of physician lifelong learning. *Journal of Continuing Medical Education, 84*(8), 1066–1074. doi:10.1097/ACM.0b013e3181acf25f

Homayounzadeh, M. (2016). Reinvestigating the determinants of lifelong learning: Can pedagogy for critical thinking contribute to developing lifelong learners? *Journal of Pedagogy and Psychology "Signum Temporis,"* 7(1), 1–14. doi:10.1515/sigtem-2016-0001

Kellenberg, F., Schmidt, J., & Werner, C. (2017). The adult learner: Self-determined, self-regulated, and reflective. *Journal of Pedagogy and Psychology "Signum Temporis,"* 9(1), 23–29. doi:10.1515/sigtem-2017-0001

Korniewicz, D. (2015). *"Application of Pat Benner's model for advanced practice practitioners," Nursing leadership and management: The advanced practice role.* Lancaster, PA: DEStech Publications, Inc.

Longworth, N. (2003). *Lifelong learning in action: Transforming education in the 21st century.* London: Kogan Page.

Lüftenegger, M., Schober, B., Van de Schoot, R., Wagner, P., Finsterwald, M., & Spiel, C. (2012). Lifelong learning as a goal – Do autonomy and self-regulation in school result in well-prepared pupils? *Learning and Instruction, 22*(1), 27–36. doi:10.1016/j.learninstruc.2011.06.001

National Organization of Nurse Practitioner Faculties. (2016). *White Paper: The Doctor of Nursing Practice Nurse Practitioner Clinical Scholar 2016 Executive Summary.* Retrieved from https://cdn.ymaws.com/www.nonpf.org/resource/resmgr/docs/AcademicPracticePartnersFina.pdf

Patra, K. (2010). *Lifelong learning or lifelong yearnings: A new design for teaching and learning.* Retrieved from https://www.inderscienceonline.com/loi/ijmie

Sigma Theta Tau. (1999). *Clinical scholarship resource paper.* Clinical Scholarship Task Force. Retrieved from https://www.sigmanursing.org/docs/default-source/position-papers/clinical_scholarship_paper.pdf?sfvrsn=4

V ANSWERS TO THE APPLICATION EXERCISES

CHAPTER 3: INSTITUTIONAL REVIEW BOARD PROCESS AND THE DNP PROJECT

Answers for Application Exercises: Preparing and Submitting an IRB Application for a DNP Project

1. The first step Sally should take to have a solid plan for preparing and submitting her DNP project IRB application is to examine the website for her university. In this case, Sally would examine the website at XYZ University, where key information is located for the IRB process and application materials. Also, there will be IRB contact information included, usually a telephone number and email addresses for key IRB staff, and personnel to provide guidance and support through the IRB process.

   It is prudent to see if the DNP project faculty/mentor and/or IRB staff and personnel will review the IRB application prior to final submission for thoroughness and accuracy. The IRB application must meet all the IRB requirements so that no changes need to be made since this may result in unavoidable delays and negatively impact on the timeline for completion of the DNP project or graduation.

2. DNP projects often involve direct contact with human subjects. For example, IRB permission is required if/when the DNP project includes any contact with a human subject including

touching, interviewing, or direct care. Some university and organizational IRB committees do not require IRB approval if the DNP project is a quality improvement project; however, the DNP graduates need to have the knowledge, skills, and competencies about the IRB process when completing a doctoral program. Many sources of contemporary literature and publishers will not publish DNP projects that have not received IRB approval. The same is true of professional presentations and some organizations that do not allow a professional paper or poster presentation if the work has not received IRB approval.

3. The purpose of the IRB is to protect human subjects involved in research. While there are multiple areas the IRB committee oversees, their main role is to review the DNP project and determine if human subjects are involved in the DNP project. When/if human subjects are involved in the DNP project, the IRB determines if the subjects are protected through application of ethical principles involved in the research process. There are risks to human subjects in every DNP project that involves human subjects. The goal of submitting the DNP project to the IRB is to be certain that the DNP project meets all requisite national standards and guidelines for human subject protection.

4. Typically, information on the IRB process for specific academic organizations like colleges and universities or healthcare organizations is located on the organization's website. For example, the academic or healthcare organization may have a site labeled IRB Information or Research. Typically, all forms needed to submit the IRB application and guidelines for completion of the IRB application are clearly labeled and available for downloading from the organization's website. The organization's website may also have a section titled *Frequently Asked Questions (FAQs)* to facilitate knowledge and understanding of the IRB application and process. The website often includes a calendar with IRB dates for submission and notification.

5. Sally will be collaborating with multiple key stakeholders and key players in both the DNP program and in the IRB office during the IRB application process. Sally should reach out to her DNP faculty/mentor when she is unsure or in doubt about any aspect of the IRB application and/or process. For example, it is human nature to share questions and concerns with a friend or colleague, and the friend or colleague can be supportive and a good listener; however, the friend or colleague may not be familiar with the specific IRB application

and processes at Sally's university. The ultimate goal for Sally is to become familiar with her university's specific IRB application and process and reach out to the IRB key personnel and staff to be sure she is submitting IRB materials in the right manner, with the right documents, to the right place, and at the right time.

6. Communication strategies Sally should consider when completing the IRB application will include email communication, telephone calls and in some cases, face-to-face meetings or video conference calls. Email stands for *electronic mail* and is the preferred communication strategy used today. One of the challenges Sally will face with email and the IRB application and process is that the IRB is a very busy office and reviews all IRB applications for everyone in the organization. The number of students and faculty conducting research will determine how quickly the IRB contact person will respond to Sally's email. Therefore, it is important to realize that responses to email communications may take a few hours, days, or weeks. This can be frustrating to Sally since she has a strict timeline to complete the DNP project. Therefore, it is important to build in extra time periods to allow for IRB waiting periods or timeline changes.

   Email is dependent on technology, and technology can sometimes fail. Therefore, it is important that Sally allow a reasonable amount of time for a response to email communications and follow up with a telephone call if she has no response in a reasonable amount of time. For example, if Sally has not received a response to an email question after 7 business days, she should call the IRB office and follow up regarding her question. The IRB website will have a person or email for communicating questions/issues, and typically they have hours of availability posted on the website as well as emergency contact information.

   When communicating with the IRB via an email, a telephone call, or a face-to-face meeting, it is important to provide a clear and succinct context for the reason and nature of your communication. For example, as the IRB is responsible for reviewing multiple research projects, it is unlikely that they will know about your specific DNP project. Therefore, it is important to prepare an overview of your project in one paragraph. Frame your question or issue in a clear and succinct manner. It is good to rehearse the conversation you plan to have with the IRB with someone who knows nothing about the IRB or to stand in front of a mirror to be certain you are clearly communicating your specific DNP project question or concern.

Sally might start by saying "Hello, my name is Sally Jones. I am a third year student in the DNP program and am currently working on completion of the IRB application for my project that involves . . . . . . My project focuses on . . . .My question is. . . .?"

7. First and foremost, Sally should revisit the IRB website and review any of the FAQs available to determine if her questions can be answered. Second, Sally could contact her faculty advisor to discuss her concerns and to obtain any additional feedback about her IRB proposal. Finally, Sally can contact a staff member at the IRB office to discuss her issue so that he or she can clarify or answer any of her questions.

8. Four common barriers/challenges Sally may experience in the IRB application process are:
   - Lack of clarity on a specific component/section of the IRB application
   - Confusion on how to follow a guideline for completion of the IRB application
   - Lack of understanding on what a specific term/word means in the IRB guidelines or on the application
   - Frustration waiting for response/approval from the IRB

9. It is perfectly normal to feel anxious with new or unfamiliar experiences like completing a DNP project and submitting an IRB application. It is important not to suppress your anxiety. Stifling or suppressing one's feelings is counterproductive and in turn often leads to elevated levels of anxiety and more counterproductive behaviors. It is important to check in with the DNP faculty advisor/mentor when feeling anxious or having self-doubt at any time in the DNP project and IRB application process.
   - Be mindful. Check in with yourself to be mindful of the important work you are doing and how this type of scholarly activity and learning is preparing you well with knowledge, skills, and competencies needed as a DNP-prepared nurse clinician or nurse executive.
   - Anxiety is fear of the unknown. It is normal to have anxiety while completing the IRB application and process as this is a new learning experience that is unfamiliar to the DNP student. It is essential to confront anxieties head on and seek out one's DNP faculty mentor/advisor for the DNP project to be sure you are on target and you have completed all necessary components of the DNP project and IRB application process.

- You want to take care of yourself during your doctoral program. This is a stressful time for many DNP students and a time you want to practice self-care. Sometimes, going for a run, exercising, or going for a walk helps one to be clear on the task and goals at hand, adding a new perspective and helping one feel calmer about the work that needs to take place to meet one's educational goals.

10. Gantt charts help the DNP student have a visual representation of the time table for realistic completion of all phases of the DNP project schedule throughout the academic year including IRB application preparation and submission. It should be noted this Gantt chart is only an example and there may be more time needed for each component of the DNP project, given the DNP student's individual circumstances. Gantt charts provide a visual portrayal of the DNP project and help the student and other key stakeholders see at a glance the progression made (or not made) toward the phases of the DNP project including the IRB application and subsequent mandatory reports that must be finalized upon completion of the DNP project. Gantt charts also facilitate a visual for the DNP student in terms of realistic due dates and activity deadlines to meet program completion. The following table from Chapter 3 is a Gantt chart example.

EXAMPLE OF GANTT CHART

	1-15-20	1-31-20	2-15-20	2-28-20	3-15-20	3-30-20
Select DNP project topic by Jan 31						
Get DNP faculty input/ feedback on DNP project topic by Jan 31			Rec'd 2/15			
Begin review of literature by Feb 1			Began 2/15			
Complete review of literature by Feb 28						

1. Enter each DNP project activity/phase with a description and outcomes
2. Highlight each of the DNP project activities or phases to correlate to the timeline on the vertical access (by week, by month, and include the year)
3. Color code each of the DNP project activities or phases to correlate to the timeline on the vertical access (by week, by month, and include the year) using the following key:

(continued)

EXAMPLE OF GANTT CHART (*CONTINUED*)

4. Green (white) = on time and no issues
5. Yellow (gray) = nearly on time and project activity/phase is moving forward with few interferences or few dependencies on others to move the project to green status
6. Red (black) = There are major holdups and or issues and this activity/phase is not moving forward or at a standstill/major impasse. This means that there are currently major threats to the project and high risk of not completing the project on time or more support is needed to move the activity/phase forward

---

More information about how to create a Gantt chart in Excel can be found at: www.template.net/tutorials/create-a-gantt-chart-in-excel

CHAPTER 4: DATA COLLECTION, MANAGEMENT, ENTRY, AND ANALYSIS

Answers for Application Exercises: Psychometric Measures, Validity, and Reliability

1. Yes, this is an appropriate psychometric test to use for this clinical event. Mr. Jacobs demonstrated clinical evidence such as forgetfulness and orientation to time (day of week) and place. The MMSE is a short cognitive mental functioning test suitable for use with older adults with signs and symptoms of dementia. It is an 11-item instrument that evaluates a person's orientation to time, place, recall ability, short-term memory, and arithmetic ability (Folstein et al., 1975).

   However, this test cannot be used to diagnose dementia but can be used to indicate cognitive impairment. Scores can be completed immediately by summing the points to each completed task with a maximum score of 30 (no impairment). The recommended cutting point used to indicate cognitive impairment deserving further investigation is 23 or 24 out of 30.

   More on This Topic
   Folstein, M., Folstein, S., & McHugh P. (1975). "Mini-Mental State" A practical method for grading the cognitive state of patients for the clinician. *Journal of Psychiatric Research, 12*, 189–198. doi:10.1016/0022-3956(75)90026-6

Harrison, J. K., Fearon, P., Noel-Storr, A. H., McShane, R., Stott, D. J., & Quinn, T. J. (2015). Informant Questionnaire on Cognitive Decline in the Elderly (IQCODE) for the diagnosis of dementia within a secondary care setting. *Cochrane Database Systematic Review, 3*, 1. doi:10.1002/14651858.CD010772.pub2

Robinson, L., Tang, E., & Taylor, J. P. (2015). Dementia: Timely diagnosis and early intervention. *BMJ, 350*, 1–6. doi:10.1136/bmj.h3029

2. The clinical evidence was clear in this case study. Mrs. Jacobs provided historical data about Mr. Jacobs's activities of daily living and Mr. Jacobs displayed a decrease in cognitive ability by his answers to queries from Terry. The examples from the case report include the following reports from Mrs. Jacobs citing examples like forgetting his keys to the car, where he parked the car, not knowing the names of his grandchildren, and often forgetting where his home was located. She further stated that he frequently would forget the day of the week or even know where the bathroom was located in his house. Mr. Jacobs could readily recall events related to his childhood but he had difficulty with knowing the day of the week or current events, such as the president of the United States, or his wife's first name. Other mental health changes that Terry noted were that Mr. Jacobs had difficulty identifying an object she would hold up and trying to count backward from 100. Finally, Terry administered the MMSE and Mr. Jacobs scored 23, which indicated cognitive impairment. The findings in the case study are consistent with findings of Naqvi et al. (2015), who provided data about the use of the MMSE in a variety of elderly patient populations. As a result of the health history obtained from Mr. and Mrs. Jacob, the evidence-based clinical literature about the use of the MMSE for cognitive impairment among elderly populations, it is clear that the use of the MMSE as a screening tool for cognitive impairment is supported.

More on This Topic

Naqvi, R. M., Haider, S., Tomlinson, G., & Alibhai, S. (2015). Cognitive assessments in multicultural populations using the Rowland Universal Dementia Assessment Scale: A systematic review and meta-analysis. *Canadian Medical Association Journal, 187*(5), E169–E175. doi:10.1503/cmaj.140802

3. The MMSE was developed by Rovner and Folstein (1987) as a screening tool for elderly patients who may display symptoms of cognitive functioning. The standard clinical diagnostic use

of the MMSE relates to the evaluation of individuals where there is concern about dementia, particularly mental health status related to cognitive functioning. Reports from Sallam and Mostafa (2013) demonstrated that when elderly patients were screened by using this tool, over 95% of patients were later worked up for physical changes associated with dementia or early-onset Alzheimer's disease dementia (ADD). However, more recently, the MMSE has been used to evaluate patients with ADD (Ahmad, Orrell, Iliffe, & Gracie, 2010). Studies by Arevalo-Rodriguez (2015) have demonstrated that the MMSE when used as an initial screening tool for cognitive impairment or symptoms associated with ADD, then clinicians are more apt to complete further neurological workup after the patient's initial clinical presentation.

More on This Topic
Ahmad, S., Orrell, M., Iliffe, S., & Gracie, A. (2010). GPs' attitudes, awareness, and practice regarding early diagnosis of dementia. *British Journal of General Practice, 60*(578), e360–e365. doi:10.3399/bjgp10X515386

Arevalo-Rodriguez, I., Smailagic, N., Roque, I. F. M., Ciapponi, A., Sanchez-Perez, E., Giannakou, A., . . . Cullum, S. (2015). Mini-Mental State Examination (MMSE) for the detection of Alzheimer's disease and other dementias in people with mild cognitive impairment (MCI). *Cochrane Database Systematic Review,* (3), 1. doi:10.1002/14651858.CD010783.pub2

Harrison, J. K., Fearon, P., Noel-Storr, A. H., McShane, R., Stott, D. J., & Quinn, T. J. (2015). Informant Questionnaire on Cognitive Decline in the Elderly (IQCODE) for the diagnosis of dementia within a secondary care setting. *Cochrane Database Systematic Review, 3*, 1. doi:10.1002/14651858.CD010772.pub2

Robinson, L., Tang, E., & Taylor, J. P. (2015). Dementia: Timely diagnosis and early intervention. *BMJ, 350*, 1–6. doi:10.1136/bmj.h3029

Rovner, B. W., & Folstein, M. F. (1987). Mini-mental state exam in clinical practice. *Hospital Practice (Off Ed), 22*(1A), 99, 103, 106, 110.

Sallam, K., & Mostafa A. M. R. (2013). The Use of the Mini-Mental State Examination and the Clock-Drawing Test for Dementia in a Tertiary Hospital. *Journal of Clinical and Diagnostic Research, 7*(3), 484–488. doi:10.7860/JCDR/2013/4203.2803

4. Folstein, Folstein, and McHugh (1975) reported test–retest reliability of the MMSE between 0.89 and 0.93, and interrater reliability has not fallen below 0.82. Furthermore, the interrater reliability gave a Pearson correlation of 0.95 and a Kendall

coefficient of 0.63 in a sample of 15 neurological patients. Moreover, Jae Baek et al. (2016) have reported the MMSE test–retest reliability to be culturally sensitive in a patient population of Koreans. The reliability of the MMSE has been well reported in a variety of patient populations that have presented in community and individual patient settings, and consistent findings have been obtained.

More on This Topic
Folstein, M., Folstein, S., & McHugh P. (1975). "Mini-Mental State" A practical method for grading the cognitive state of patientsfor the clinician. *Journal of Psychiatric Research, 12*, 189–198. doi:10.1016/0022-3956(75)90026-6

Jae Baek, M., Kim, K., Park, Y., & Kim, S. (2016). The Validity and Reliability of the Mini Mental State Examination-2 for Detecting Mild Cognitive Impairment and Alzheimer's Disease in a Korean Population. *PLoS One, 11*(9). doi:10.1371/journal.pone.0163792

Mitchell, A. J., & Malladi, S. (2010) Screening and case-finding tools for the detection of dementia. Part II: evidence-based meta-analysis of single-domain tests. *The American Journal of Geriatric Psychiatry, 18*(9), 783–800. doi:10.1097/JGP.0b013e3181cdecd6

NICE Pathways. (2016). *Dementia diagnosis and assessment* (p. 10). Retrieved from https://www.nice.org.uk/about/what-we-do/our-programmes/about-nice-pathways

5. Initially, the MMSE demonstrated validity with a small sample of elderly patients (Folstein, Anthony, Parhad, Duffy, & Gruenberg, 1985). The MMSE correlated 0.78 with the Wechsler Adult Intelligence Scale (WAIS) Verbal IQ scale. Predictive validity: it was found by Mitrushina and Satz (1994) in a small study that those whose scores decreased by more than seven points in 3 years were diagnosed with neurological deficits. Several clinicians have compared the MMSE with other cognitive impairment measures such as the clinical dementia rating scale (CDR: -0.82, $p = .000$; Babacan-Yildiz et al., 2016) and (CDR: .56–.83; Jae Baek et al., 2016). There are clear evidence-based clinical guidelines that recommend the use of the MMSE as a screening tool to assess cognitive impairment in elderly patients.

More on This Topic
Babacan-Yıldız, G., Ur-Özçelik, E., Kolukısa, M., Işık AT, Gürsoy E, Kocaman G, Çelebi A. (2016). [Validity and Reliability Studies of Modified Mini Mental State Examination (MMSE-E) For Turkish Illiterate Patients With Diagnosis of Alzheimer Disease]. *Turk Psikiyatri Derg, 27*(1):41–46.

Folstein, M., Anthony, J. C., Parhad, I., Duffy, B., & Gruenberg, E. M. (1985). The meaning of cognitive impairment in the elderly. *Journal of the American Geriatrics Society, 33*(4), 228–235. doi:10.1111/j.1532-5415.1985.tb07109.x

Lacy, M., Kaemmerer, T., & Czipri, S. (2014). Standardized Mini-Mental State Examination Scores and Verbal Memory Performance at a Memory Center. *American Journal of Alzheimer's Disease and Other Dementias, 30*(2), 145–152. doi:10.1177/1533317514539378

Mitchell, A. J. (2017). The Mini-Mental State Examination (MMSE): An update on its diagnostic validity for cognitive disorders. In A. J. Larner (Ed.), *Chapter 3: Cognitive screening instruments: A practical approach* (pp. 15–46). London: Springer-Verlag.

Mitrushina, M., & Satz, P. (1994). Utility of mini-mental state examination in assessing cognition in the elderly. *Aging (Milano), 6*(6), 427–432.

6. The MMSE can be scored immediately with a total score of 30. The questions can be scored immediately by summing the points to each completed task with a maximum score of 30 (no impairment). It is recommended to treat unanswered questions as errors (Folstein et al., 1975).

More on This Topic

Creavin, S. T., Wisniewski, S., Noel-Storr, A. H., Trevelyan, C. M., Hampton, T., Rayment, D., . . . Cullum, S. (2016). Mini-Mental State Examination (MMSE) for the detection of dementia in clinically unevaluated people aged 65 and over in community and primary care populations. *Cochrane Database of Systematic Reviews.* doi:10.1002/14651858.CD011145.pub2

Folstein, M., Folstein, S., & McHugh P. (1975). "Mini-Mental State" A practical method for grading the cognitive state of patients for the clinician. *Journal of Psychiatric Research, 12*, 189–198. doi:10.1016/0022-3956(75)90026-6

Gao, M. Y., Yang, M., Kuang, W. H., & Qiu, P. Y. (2015). Factors and validity analysis of Mini- Mental State Examination in Chinese elderly people. *Journal of Peking University, Health Sciences, 47*(3), 443–449.

7. Based on Mr. Jacobs's initial score of 23, this would be interpreted as having increased odds of dementia. This score may be consistent with Mr. Jacobs's age, memory loss, and activities of daily living. Because of this score, it would be appropriate to refer Mr. Jacobs to a geriatrician and neurologist for further workup for dementia. Additionally,

he would need further workup to rule out any differential diagnosis for cognitive decline such as hypothyroidism, diabetes, parkinsonian syndrome, and cardiovascular disorders.

More on This Topic

Om, P., & Shailesh, S. (2016). Differential diagnosis for cognitive decline in the elderly. *Journal of Geriatric Mental Health,* *3*(1), 21–28. Retrieved from http://www.jgmh.org/article. asp?issn=2348-9995;year=2016;volume=3;issue=1;spage=21;epa ge=28;aulast=Prakash

8. Nurse practitioners can use the MMSE as a general screening tool with elderly patients who present with symptoms associated with changes in cognitive function. The specific areas of cognitive functioning should include an abnormal score on the MMSE as well as the patient's ability to systematically answer questions associated with memory loss, activities of daily living, and ability to interpret simple reading examples.

More on This Topic

Brent, S., & Hartmann, B. (2011). Evaluation of suspected dementia. *American Family Physician, 84*(8), 895–902.

Cooper, C., Sommerlad, A., Lyketsos, C. G., & Livingston, G. (2015). Modifiable predictors of dementia in mild cognitive impairment: A systematic review and meta-analysis. *American Journal of Psychiatry, 172,* 323–333. doi:10.1176/appi. ajp.2014.14070878

9. Since the MMSE was developed to provide data about cognitive impairment in older adults, it would be best to use the MMSE as an annual screening tool in elderly patient populations in ages above 50 years. Because the MMSE is an easy clinical assessment tool and provides a score for general cognitive impairment, patient scores could be compared annually. Comparison of annual MMSE scores would provide data about cognitive changes that may occur in patients as they age.

More on This Topic

Eshkoor, S. A., Hamid, T. A., Mun, C. Y., & Ng, C. K. (2015). Mild cognitive impairment and its management in older people. *Clinical Interventions in Aging, 10,* 687–693. doi:10.2147/CIA. S73922

Langa, K. M., & Levine, D. A. (2014). The diagnosis and management of mild cognitive impairment: A clinical review. *JAMA, 312,* 2551–2561. doi:10.1001/jama.2014.13806

10. Depending on when the MMSE has been administered, there may be changes to the MMSE. It is best to compare scores from the MMSE annually since cognitive impairment occurs as one ages. Perhaps, the MMSE scores may significantly provide clinical information on elderly patients who are being evaluated for cognitive impairment. Cognitive changes in elderly patients occur over time; thus, annual use of the MMSE would provide data about the patient's cognitive ability over time.

More on This Topic

Trzepacz, P. T., Hochstetler, H., Wang, S., Walker, B., Saykin, A. J., & Alzheimer's Disease Neuroimaging Initiative. (2015). Relationship between the Montreal Cognitive Assessment and Mini-mental State Examination for assessment of mild cognitive impairment in older adults. *BMC Geriatrics, 15,* 107. doi:10.1186/s12877-015-0103-3

Vega, J. N., & Newhouse, P. A. (2014). Mild cognitive impairment: diagnosis, longitudinal course, and emerging treatments. *Current Psychiatry Reports, 16,* 490. doi:10.1007/s11920-014-0490-8

CHAPTER 6: TEAM BUILDING, INTERPROFESSIONAL COLLABORATION

Answers for Application Exercises: Team Building, Leadership, and Interprofessional Collaboration

Part I: Suggested answers for understanding overall IPEC competencies, subcategories, and exemplars from the case study.

IPEC Core Competency	IPEC Subcategories	Case Study Exemplars
Competency 1: Values/Ethics for Interprofessional Practice	VE2–VE4 VE5–VE10	Hispanic immigrant, feel welcomed, bilingual volunteer NP Hazel asks Maria to stay during history and physical

(continued)

IPEC Core Competency	IPEC Subcategories	Case Study Exemplars
Competency 2: Roles/ Responsibilities	RR1 RR2 RR5 RR7	Introduction to Mr. Garzon Keeps Maria in room to communicate Discusses treatment and plan of care Follow-up plan explained
Competency 3: Interprofessional Communication	CC1–CC4 CC8	Bilingual staff member Follow-up plan
Competency 4: Teams and Teamwork	TT1–TT3 TT5–TT7 TT11	Engages volunteer, bilingual All HC personnel engaged to provide care Teamwork evident

HC, healthcare.

Part II: Suggested answers for general questions providing exemplars (a–m) and using the IPEC competencies and subcategories.

1. How would you plan healthcare for a transient patient population? Apply the IPEC competencies and subcategories to your answer.
   a. Understand the needs of the population
   b. Sources for getting needs met
   c. Understand relationship between homelessness and health
   d. Consider relationship between hospital and clinic staff
   e. Provide for partnerships with community providers serving homeless (share staff)
   f. Develop methods to share data (both ways, if possible)
   g. Set up provider and pharmacy networks
   h. Institute ways to eliminate or limit out-of-pocket costs
   i. Educate medical and social work staff on EBPs (especially, as they pertain to homeless/high-need patients)
   j. Provide options for medical respite programs and linkages to supportive housing
   k. Obtain funding from any community or private benefit funds to help meet the needs of patients
   l. Document homelessness in the medical electronic record for data collection

Suggested application of the IPEC competencies for the aforementioned examples:

IPEC Core Competency	IPEC Subcategories and Exemplars
Competency 1: Values/Ethics for Interprofessional Practice	VE1 a, j VE2 d, j VE3 a, j VE4 e, j VE5 b, e VE6 c, d VE7 b, c, f, g VE8 c, f, g, k VE9 k VE10 h, i, l, m
Competency 2: Roles/ Responsibilities	RR1 a, e, f, j RR2 b, e, f, j, k RR3 c, d, e, f RR4 d, e, f, j RR5 c, d, e, f, j RR6 e, f, g, j, k RR7 e, f, g, j, k RR8 e, f, j RR9 e, f, j, l RR10 e, f, h, i, j, l, m

IPEC Core Competency	IPEC Subcategories and Exemplars
Competency 3: Interprofessional Communication	CC1 a, c, e, f, j CC2 a, c, e, f, j CC3 a, b, c, e, f, j CC4 a, b, c, e, f, j CC5 a, c, e, f, j CC6 a, c, e, f, j CC7 a, b, c, d, e, f, g, j CC8 a, c, d, e, f, g, h, i, j, k, l, m
Competency 4: Teams and Teamwork	TT1 a, c, d, e, f, j TT2 a, c, d, e, f, j TT3 a, c, d, e, f, i, j, l TT4 a, e, f, j, k, l TT5 a, b, e, f, j TT6 a, e, f, j TT7 a, b, c, e, f, g, j, m TT8 a, e, f, g, j, m TT9 a, b, c, e, f, g, j, k TT10 a, d, e, f, g, j TT11 a, d, e, f, g, h, j

2. What steps would you take to address the cultural needs of a patient population?
   - Language appropriate patient education brochures
   - Signage available to include multiple cultural groups
   - Workforce diversity to include healthcare staff consistent with population being served
   - Ongoing training of staff about cultural awareness
   - Form partnerships with local communities, churches, other healthcare services that provide healthcare benefits to the patient population
   - Develop outcome measures consistent with specific performance of healthcare workers who meet the needs of the population
   - Align services consistent with patient preferences
   - Locate the healthcare facility within the community that serves the population
   - Provide healthcare data consistent with cultural needs of patient population for all community to review and have input
   - Provide educational sessions for patients in preferred language of population

3. Discuss the systemic changes needed to provide effective quality patient care.
   - Develop shared vision among all healthcare agencies to serve homeless population
   - Partner with community providers serving homeless (share staff)
   - Share data (among all agencies, if possible)
   - Ensure provider and pharmacy networks are in sync
   - Eliminate/limit out-of-pocket costs (if possible)
   - Train medical and social work staff on EBPs (especially as they pertain to homeless/high-need patients)
   - Develop/expand medical respite programs and linkages to supportive housing
   - Use hospital community benefit funds to help meet patient needs
   - Plan referral processes that are cost-effective
   - Implement evaluation plan that involves all key stakeholders
   - Provide patient representation on committees or evaluation processes

- Develop supplement funding opportunities or budgets consistent with meeting the needs of the population
- Provide annual reports related to service provisions for this population within the community
- Document homelessness in your electronic health record
- Set up website consistent with the shared vision and if possible for data collection related to healthcare services provided among the constituents

More on This Topic

Agency for Healthcare Research and Quality. (2018). TeamSTEPPS Team Strategies and Tools to Enhance Performance and Patient Safety. Retrieved from http://teamstepps.ahrq.gov

Centers for Disease Control and Prevention. (2018). Testing for Tuberculosis (TB). Retrieved from http://www.cdc.gov/tb/publications/factsheets/testing/tb_factsheet.pdf

Institute of Healthcare Improvement Open School Online Courses. (2015). Retrieved from http://app.ihi.org/lms/onlinelearning.aspx

Nahid, P., Dorman, S. E., Alipanah, N., Barry, P. M., Brozek, J. L., Cattamanchi, A., . . . Vernon, A. (2016). Official American Thoracic Society/Centers for Disease Control and Prevention/Infectious Diseases Society of America Clinical Practice Guidelines: Treatment of Drug-Susceptible Tuberculosis. *Clinical Infectious Diseases, 63*, e147. doi:10.1093/cid/ciw376

The U.S. Department of Housing and Urban Development, Office of Community Planning and Development. (2013). The 2013 Annual Homeless Assessment Report (AHAR) to Congress. Retrieved from https://www.onecpd.info/resources/documents/AHAR-2013-Part1.pdf

CHAPTER 8: INTERPRETATION OF FINDINGS AND IMPACT ON CLINICAL PRACTICE

Answers for Application Exercises: Quantitative Versus Qualitative Data Methods

Exercise 1: Answers to 10-item quiz in Box 8.2

1. Answer: a
2. Answer: a
3. Answer: b

4. Answer: a
5. Answer: b
6. Answer: a
7. Answer: a
8. Answer: b
9. Answer: c
10. Answer: a

Exercise 2: Focused Interview Guide
A grounded theory approach to qualitative research methods allows the researcher to direct the focus of the research specifically in the direction of the phenomenon of study, in this case the concept of pain. A focused interview guide may be used to obtain information about the pain that is experienced by the participants. The focused interview guide may assist the researcher in obtaining any themes, patterns of behavior, or attitudes about pain. It would be important to provide questions about pain that directly impact on the care of the patient. In the case study provided, the development of open-ended questions associated with the variables that describe Mrs. Smith's experience with pain would be essential content that would need to be considered. It is best to ask questions that cannot be obtained directly from the medical record such as the patient's age and diagnosis. An example of a focused interview guide may include questions such as:

1. Describe the type of pain that you are experiencing.
2. Can you tell me about the intensity of the pain?
3. What makes the pain better?
4. What makes the pain worse?
5. Do you experience any emotional changes when you have the pain?
6. What do you understand as the cause of the pain?
7. Are you aware of the pain medication that you are taking?
8. Do you feel that the pain medication is helping you cope with the pain?
9. How would you change your pain treatment plan?
10. Has your family helped you cope with the pain?

The variables (patient's descriptive experience, sensory and emotional descriptors, treatment, coping) associated with the individual's pain experience have been considered in the focused interview guide as follows:

Variable	Item Number
Pain experience	1–4
Emotional changes	5
Cause of pain	6
Treatment	7–9
Family and coping	10

The example used for the preceding *focused interview guide* can be expanded to include a variety of other variables associated with pain. For example, the "pain items" could be refocused to include more general or more specific descriptors depending on which direction the researcher may be interested in exploring.

Exercise 3: Critique of a Quantitative Research Project
Suggested answers for the guidelines used to determine if the quantitative research methods used for this study answered the research question:

- *Does the research question imply a relationship between the independent and dependent variables?* First, identify the research question: "This study was conducted to determine whether bacteriophage ØX174 could penetrate used vinyl and latex examination gloves after standardized manipulations." Second, review the research question and readily determine the independent and dependent variables for this study. An independent variable is defined as the manipulated (or treatment) variable; in experimental research, it is the variable that can cause or influence the dependent variable (Creswell & Plano Clark, 2011) while a dependent variable is defined as the outcome variable of interest, the variable hypothesized, to depend on or be caused by another variable (independent); see Creswell and Plano Clark (2011). For this study, the dependent variables are the gloves (vinyl or latex) whereas the independent variable would be the standardized hand manipulations.
- *Is the research question clearly stated?* Yes, the research question was clearly stated as: "This study was conducted to determine whether bacteriophage ØX174 could penetrate used vinyl and latex examination gloves after standardized manipulations."
- *Is there an intervention or treatment suggested?* Yes, the intervention has been defined as a standardized method of hand manipulations designed to mimic patient care activities performed on groups of gloves in advance of testing.

- *What type of research design was described?* This was an experimental study conducted in a laboratory setting. Although the manuscript did not specifically identify the type of research design, it was assumed since the study was conducted in a basic microbiology laboratory.
- *Are the methods clearly described (e.g., sample, procedures for the study, treatment or nontreatment groups)?* Yes, the procedures were clearly written specifically for the manipulation of the gloves as well as the specific laboratory procedures that were used to test each glove pair. This was evidenced by the narrative components under the subheadings "procedures of glove manipulations" and "preparation and assay of phage."
- *What types of comparisons are made and do these comparisons provide support for the independent and dependent variables of the study?* Yes, there are several comparisons between the types of gloves (latex or vinyl), levels of manipulations (0–3), and type of leak (viral, visible, not visible).
- *Were the data collection procedures described?* Yes, all data collection procedures were clearly described. The total number of examination gloves (240 vinyl and 240 latex) was tested with 60 each in the four categories. The sample size was adequate since the sensitivity of the laboratory testing was enough to determine a difference between the type of gloves as well as the leakage rate for each type (latex or vinyl) of glove.
- *Was the data collected appropriate for the study?* Yes, it was an experimental laboratory study that was completed to determine viral leakage rates between vinyl and latex gloves.

More on This Topic
Creswell, J. W. (2014). *Research design: Qualitative, quantitative, and mixed-methods approaches*. Thousand Oaks, CA: Sage Publications.
Creswell, J. W., & Plano Clark, V. L. (2011). *Designing and conducting mixed methods research*. Thousand Oaks, CA, Sage Publications.
Glogowska, M. (2011). Paradigms, pragmatism and possibilities: Mixed-methods research in speech and language therapy. *International Journal of Language Communication Disorders, 46,* 251–260. doi:10.3109/13682822.2010.507614
Scammon, D. L., Tomoaia-Cotisel, A., Day, R. L., Day, J., Kim, J., Waitzman, N. J., . . . Magill, M. K. (2013). Connecting the dots and merging meaning: Using mixed methods to study primary care delivery transformation. *Health Services Research, 48,* 2181–2207. doi:10.1111/1475-6773.12114

Strauss, A., & Corbin, J. (1998). *Basic qualitative research* (2nd ed.). Thousand Oaks, CA: Sage Publications.

Van den Bruel, A., Jones, C., Thompson, M., & Mant, D. (2016). C-reactive protein point-of-care testing in acutely ill children: a mixed methods study in primary care. *Archives of Disease in Childhood, 10*, 1136.

Walsh, D., & Evans, K. (2014). Critical realism: An important theoretical perspective for midwifery research. *Midwifery, 30*, e1–e6. doi:10.1016/j.midw.2013.09.002

Zhang, W., & Creswell, J. (2013). The use of "mixing" procedure of mixed methods in health services research. *Medical Care, 51*, e51–e57. doi:10.1097/MLR.0b013e31824642fd

CHAPTER 9: DISSEMINATION OF FINDINGS, PRESENTATIONS, AND PUBLICATIONS

Answers for Application Exercises: Development of a Meaningful Poster Presentation

1. The first step that Susie should undertake is to obtain a copy of the purpose of the conference and the review committee's guidelines associated with poster presentations. The conference purpose will determine topic areas that will be presented while the poster guidelines will provide guidance as to the abstract submission, size of the poster, word count, and expectations of the presenter. Once Susie reads the guidelines, she will be able to develop her content consistent with the expectations of the conference review committee members.

2. Yes, since this provides opportunities for staff to become familiar with presentations for professional meetings. Additionally, this will provide learning opportunities for the staff as well as peer-review processes that will help to further develop the content area. Often, other clinical staff members who were involved in the data collection process of the project and/or contributed to staff presentations may provide added insight into the discussion or recommendation section of the poster presentation. One recommendation for lifelong learning includes the use of peer review as a method to enhance one's professional growth. Therefore, by having others being involved in a poster presentation may enhance one's ability to grow as a clinical scholar.

3. Poster presentations are excellent opportunities to network with colleagues and showcase one's clinical scholarship. Often,

poster presentations provide opportunities to discuss findings with colleagues who have similar interests and who may assist in similar future projects. By having the opportunity to discuss the content of the poster with attendees who read the poster and ask questions about the content enables taking information back to your organization or their organization. Often, presenters provide a one-page handout about their poster so that attendees can contact them for future networking opportunities.

4. The poster information should be located under the "call for abstracts" for the conference. Most professional organizations provide detailed guidelines as to where, how, or when to submit for a poster presentation. Often, submission of poster presentations need to be completed via an "online" format and applicants will be directed to a website that will be used for submission. It is important to follow the submission guidelines specifically developed for the conference so that the poster is not rejected for technical issues.

5. Most professional conferences have similar components that will need to be addressed by the poster presenters. Since the poster presentation is a summary of your project, it needs to be concise and in a format that is readily available and easy to read. In general, the areas that will need to be addressed include:

   • Abstract
   • Overall objectives of the project
   • Methods
   • Findings/Results
   • Conclusions/Recommendations

   The overall headings of the project should include the title (according to number of characters allowed), type of project (research, evidence-based quality assurance), authors or contributors (include all individuals who contributed to the project, listing the principal investigator first and then all others next), and organization (university, hospital system, or another healthcare organization). Finally, it is important to design the poster in an aesthetically pleasing manner so that the conference participants can easily read your poster and contribute insight into your area of expertise.

6. Susie can overcome her anxiety in several ways. One of the easiest ways to overcome her anxiety is to attend a local professional meeting and view other poster presentations, network with colleagues at that meeting, and review how

others present their data. A second way includes discussion with her peers in the DNP program, DNP program faculty, and other clinical staff who have had opportunities to present at professional meetings. Often, discussion with colleagues can provide insight as to the positive and negative experiences that may occur during the preparation and presentation of a poster. A third method to decrease Susie's anxiety may be to complete a "mock review" of her draft poster. A "mock review" basically is presentation of the poster to a group of graduate students, clinical staff, or other healthcare providers who are interested in the clinical topic. This will provide an opportunity for Susie to practice how she will respond to questions as well as obtain feedback about the clarity of the written components the poster. Using some or all of these techniques will help Susie cope with her own anxiety associated with the presentation, preparation, and submission of the poster. Additionally, Susie will gain more confidence and become more knowledgeable about participating in professional conferences.

7. As a result of successfully completing a poster presentation, Susie will grow professionally in several ways. For example, because this process is a peer-reviewed exercise, Susie will become more confident in her ability to present clinical findings to others interested in the topic. Second, she will be able to teach others how to prepare for professional presentations as well as provide feedback for improvement. Third, Susie will be able to meet other healthcare providers interested in her topic and develop professional relationships associated with other projects and/or presentations. Finally, Susie will be able to become more of a clinical scholar by asking future research or evidence-based practice questions that will trigger others to work with her and have opportunities to further develop the topic area.

8. Most professional conferences have developed evaluation criteria for acceptance of a poster presentation. It is important to review the evaluation criteria at the outset or when reviewing the conference purpose and "call for abstracts." Often the evaluation criteria may include the following areas:
   • Adherence to submission instructions
   • Adherence to ethical standards
   • Clarity of abstract
   • Soundness of methods used for the project
   • Completeness of the project such as supporting evidence
   • Presentation of the results and accuracy of statistical analysis

- Overall aesthetics of the design of the poster presentation

The criteria for evaluating a poster presentation are dependent on the type of professional conference, the conference review committee members' recommendations, and the type of sponsoring organization.

More on This Topic

Christenbery, T. L., & Latham, T. G. (2013). Creating effective scholarly posters: A guide for DNP students. *Journal of the American Academy of Nurse Practitioners*, 25(1), 16–23. doi:10.1111/j.1745-7599.2012.00790.x

Gundogan, B., Koshy, K., Kurar, L., & Whitehurst, K. (2019). How to make an academic poster. *Annals of Medicine and Surgery, 11,* 69–71. doi:10.1016/j.amsu.2016.09.001

Miller, J. E. (2007). Preparing and presenting effective research posters. *Health Services Research, 42,* 311–328. doi:10.1111/j.1475-6773.2006.00588.x

INDEX

abstract conceptualization, Kolb's learning theory, 123
accommodating, learning theory, 126
active experimentation, Kolb's learning theory, 123
aligned interests, 108
American Hospital Association (AHA), 17
American Organization of Nurse Executives (AONE), 17
assent process, 40–41
assimilating, learning theory, 126
authorship, 159

Bandura's Self-Efficacy Theory, 101
Beck's Depression Inventory (BDI) scale, 67
Benner's Model for Advanced Practice Practitioners, 183–185
biophysiological measures, 68–69
bivariate analyses, 73

"call for abstracts," 164–168
categorical variables, 74
CITI program. *See* Collaborative Institutional Training Initiative program
clinical environment

action plan and timeline, 87
challenges, 87
design quality, 86
evidence-based healthcare designs, 86
physical environments, 86–87
clinical findings
critical evaluation, 148
data interpretation, 149
evidence-based clinical inquiry, 147
expertise, 148
initial clinical question, 146
reflective practice, 148
reviewing, 148
"so what" questions, 147
clinical journal publication, 193
clinical scholarship
clinical question, 187–188
clinical scholars, 186–187, 192–194
Clinical Scholarship Task Force, 186
competencies, 188–189
definition, 186
evidence-based practice models, 189
lifelong-learning, 190–191
novice clinical scholar, 187
road map for, 188, 191–192
Clinical Scholarship Task Force, 186